Evidence-based Clinical Chinese Medicine

Volume 2

Psoriasis Vulgaris

Evidence-based Clinical Chinese Medicine

Co Editors-in-Chief:

Charlie Changli Xue
RMIT University, Australia

Chuanjian Lu
Guangdong Provincial Hospital of Chinese Medicine, China

Volume 2
Psoriasis Vulgaris

Lead Authors:

Claire Shuiqing Zhang

Jingjie Yu

World Scientific

NEW JERSEY · LONDON · SINGAPORE · BEIJING · SHANGHAI · HONG KONG · TAIPEI · CHENNAI · TOKYO

Published by

World Scientific Publishing Co. Pte. Ltd.

5 Toh Tuck Link, Singapore 596224

USA office: 27 Warren Street, Suite 401-402, Hackensack, NJ 07601

UK office: 57 Shelton Street, Covent Garden, London WC2H 9HE

Library of Congress Cataloging-in-Publication Data

Names: Xue, Charlie Changli, author. | Lu, Chuan-jian, 1964–   author.

Title: Evidence-based clinical Chinese medicine / Charlie Changli Xue, Chuanjian Lu.

Description: New Jersey : World Scientific, 2016. | Includes bibliographical references and index.

Identifiers: LCCN 2015030389| ISBN 9789814723084 (v. 1 : hardcover : alk. paper) |

   ISBN 9789814723091 (v. 1 : paperback : alk. paper) |

   ISBN 9789814723121 (v. 2 : hardcover : alk. paper) |

   ISBN 9789814723138 (v. 2 : paperback : alk. paper) |

   ISBN 9789814759045 (v. 3 : hardcover : alk. paper) |

   ISBN 9789814759052 (v. 3 : paperback : alk. paper)

Subjects: | MESH: Medicine, Chinese Traditional--methods. | Clinical Medicine--methods. |

   Evidence-Based Medicine--methods. | Psoriasis. | Pulmonary Disease, Chronic Obstructive.

Classification: LCC RC81 | NLM WB 55.C4 | DDC 616--dc23

LC record available at http://lccn.loc.gov/2015030389

British Library Cataloguing-in-Publication Data

A catalogue record for this book is available from the British Library.

Purpose of the Monograph

This book is intended for clinicians, researchers and educators. It can be used to inform tertiary education and clinical practice by providing systematic, multi-dimensional assessments of the best available evidence for using Chinese medicine to manage each common clinical condition.

How to Use This Monograph

Some Definitions

A glossary is included, containing terms and definitions which frequently appear in the book. It also describes the definitions of statistical tests, methodological terms, evaluation tools and interventions. For example, in this book, Integrative Medicine refers to the combined use of a Chinese medicine treatment with conventional medical management, and that Combination Therapies refers to two or more Chinese medicines from different therapy groups (Chinese herbal medicine, acupuncture or other Chinese medicine therapies) administered together.

Data Analysis and Interpretation of Results

In order to synthesise the clinical evidence, a range of statistical analysis approaches are used. In general, the effect size for dichotomous data is reported as a risk ratio (RR) with 95% confidence intervals (CI), and for continuous data, they are reported as mean difference (MD) with 95%CI. Statistically significant effects are indicated with an asterisk*. Readers should note that statistically significant does not necessarily correspond with a clinically important effect. Interpretation of results should take into consideration of clinical significance, quality of studies (expressed as high, low or unclear risk of bias in this book) and heterogeneity amongst the studies. Tests for heterogeneity are conducted using the I^2 statistic. An I^2

score greater than 50% was considered to indicate substantial heterogeneity.

Use of Evidence in Practice

The Grading of Recommendations Assessment, Development and Evaluation (GRADE) approach was used to summarise the quality of evidence and results of the strength of evidence for critical and important comparisons and outcomes. Due to the diverse nature of Chinese medicine practice, treatment recommendations are not included with the summary of findings tables. Therefore readers will need to interpret the evidence with reference to the local practice environment.

Limitations

Readers should note some of the methodological limitations on classical literature and clinical evidence.

- Search terms used to search the Zhong Hua Yi Dian database may not include all terms that have been used for the condition, which may alter the findings.
- Chinese language has changed over time. Citations have been interpreted for analysis, and such interpretations may be subject to disagreement.
- Chinese medicine theory has evolved over time. As such, concepts described in classical Chinese medical literature may no longer be found in contemporary works.
- Symptoms described in citations may be common to many conditions, and a judgment was required to determine the likelihood of the citation being related to the condition. This may have introduced some bias due to the subjective nature of the judgment.
- The vast majority of the clinical evidence for Chinese medicine treatments has come from China. The applicability of the findings to other populations and other countries requires further assessment.

- Many studies included participants with varying disease severity. Where possible, subgroup analyses were undertaken to examine the effects in different sub-populations. As this was not always possible, the findings may be limited to the population included, and not to sub-populations.
- The potential risk of bias found in many included studies suggested methodological limitations. The findings for GRADE assessments based on studies of very low to moderate quality evidence should be interpreted accordingly.
- Nine major English and Chinese language databases were searched to identify clinical studies, in addition to clinical trial registers. Other studies may exist which were not identified through searches, and which may alter the findings.
- The calculation of frequency of herbal formula use was based on formula names only. It is possible that studies evaluated herbal treatments with the same or similar herb ingredients, but which were given different formula names. Due to the complexity of herbal formulas, it was considered not appropriate to make a judgment as to the similarity of formulas for analysis. As such, the frequency of formulas reported in Chapter 5 may be underestimated.
- The most frequent utilised herbs which may have contributed to the treatment effect have been described in Chapter 5. These herbs may provide leads for further exploration. Calculation of the herbs with potential effect is based on frequency of formulae reported in the studies, and doesn't take into consideration the clinical implications and functions of every herb in a formula.

Disclaimer

The information in this monograph is based on systematic analyses of the best available evidence for Chinese medicine interventions both historical and contemporary. Every effort has been made to ensure accuracy and completeness of the data of this publication. This book is intended for clinicians, researchers and educators. The practice of evidence-based medicine consists of consideration of the best available evidence, practitioners' clinical experience and judgment, and patients' preference. Not all interventions are acceptable in all countries. It is important to note that some of the substances mentioned in this book may no longer be in use, may be toxic, or be prohibited or restricted under the provisions of the Convention on International Trade in Endangered Species of Wild Fauna and Flora (CITES). Practitioners, researchers and educators are advised to comply with relevant regulations. Patients should seek professional advice from their qualified Chinese medicine practitioners.

Foreword

Since the late 20th Century, Chinese medicine, including acupuncture and herbal medicine, has been increasingly used throughout the world. The parallel development and spread of evidence-based medicine has provided challenges and opportunities for Chinese medicine.

The opportunities have been evidence-based medicine's emphasis on the effective use of the best available clinical evidence, incorporating the clinicians' clinical experience, subject to patients' preference. Such practices have a patient focus which reflects the historical nature of Chinese medicine practice. However, the challenges are also significant due to the fact that, despite the long-term development and very rich literature accumulated over 2000 years, there is an overall lack of high level clinical evidence for many of the interventions used in Chinese medicine.

To address this knowledge gap, we need to generate clinical evidence through high quality clinical studies and to evaluate evidence to enable effective use of such available evidence to promote the evidence-based Chinese medicine practice.

Modern Chinese medicine is rooted in its classical literature and the legacies of ancient doctors, grounded in practice of expert clinicians and increasingly informed by clinical and experimental research efforts. In recognition of the unique features of Chinese medicine, for each of the conditions in this series a "Whole Evidence" approach is used to provide a synthesis of different types and levels of evidence to enable practitioners to make clinical decisions informed by the current best evidence.

There are four main components of this "Whole Evidence" approach. Firstly, we present the current approaches to the diagnosis, differentiation and treatment of each condition based on expert consensus of textbooks and clinical guidelines. This provides an overview of how the condition is currently managed. The second section provides an analysis of the condition in a historical context based on systematic searches of the Zhong Hua Yi Dian, which includes the full texts of more than 1000 classical medical books. These analyses provide objective views on how the condition has been treated over two millennia, reveal continuities and discontinuities between traditional and modern practice, and suggest avenues for future research.

The third component is the assessment of evidence derived from modern clinical studies of Chinese medicine interventions. The methods established by the Cochrane Collaboration are used for conducting systematic reviews and undertaking meta-analyses of outcome data for randomised controlled trials (RCTs). In addition, the clinical relevance of meta-analysis data is enhanced by examining the herbal formulae, individual herbs and acupuncture treatments that were assessed in the RCTs and the evidence base is broadened by the inclusion of data from non-randomised, controlled clinical trials and non-controlled studies. The fourth component is to determine how the herbal medicine interventions may achieve the effects indicated by the clinical trials. Thus for each of the most frequently used herbs we provide reviews of their effects in pre-clinical models and their likely mechanisms of action.

For each condition, this "Whole Evidence" approach links clinical expertise, historical precedent, clinical research data and experimental research to provide the reader with assessments of the current state of the evidence of efficacy and safety for Chinese medicine interventions using herbal medicines, acupuncture and moxibustion and other health care practices such as *taichi*.

Since these books are available in Chinese and English, they can benefit patients, practitioners and educators internationally and enable practitioners to make clinical decisions informed by the current best evidence.

These publications represent a major milestone in Chinese medicine development and make a significant contribution to the evidence-based Chinese medicine development globally.

Co-Editors-in-Chief

Professor Charlie Changli Xue
RMIT University
Australia

Professor Chuanjian Lu
Guangdong Provincial Hospital of Chinese Medicine
China

Related Publications

1. Yu JJ, Zhang CS, Zhang AL, May B, Xue CC, Lu C. Add-on effect of Chinese herbal medicine bath to phototherapy for psoriasis vulgaris: a systematic review. *Evid Based Complement Altern Med* 2013;**2013**: 673078. doi: 10.1155/2013/673078. Epub 2013 Jul 25.
2. Zhang CS, Yu JJ, Parker S, Zhang AL, May B, Lu C, Xue CC. Oral Chinese herbal medicine combined with pharmacotherapy for psoriasis vulgaris: a systematic review. *Int J Dermatol* 2014 Nov;**53**(11): 1305–18. doi: 10.1111/ijd.12607. Epub 2014 Sep 10.
3. Parker S, Zhang AL, Zhang CS, Goodman G, Wen Z, Lu C, Xue CC. Oral granulated Chinese herbal medicine (YXBCM01) plus topical calcipotriol for psoriasis vulgaris: study protocol for a double-blind, randomized placebo controlled trial. *Trials* 2014 Dec 19;**15**:495. doi: 10.1186/1745-6215-15-495.
4. Coyle M, Deng J, Zhang AL, Yu J, Guo X, Xue CC, Lu C. Acupuncture therapies for psoriasis vulgaris: a systematic review of randomized controlled trials. *Forsch Komplementmed* 2015; **22**: 102–109.
5. Deng S, May BH, Zhang AL, Lu C, Xue CC. Phytotherapy in the management of psoriasis: a review of the efficacy and safety of oral interventions and the pharmacological actions of the main plants. *Arch Dermatol Res* 2014 Apr;**306**(3):211–29. doi: 10.1007/s00403-013-1428-4. Epub 2013 Nov 20.
6. Deng S, May BH, Zhang AL, Lu C, Xue CC. Plant extracts for the topical management of psoriasis: a systematic review and meta-analysis. *Br J Dermatol* 2013 Oct;**169**(4):769–82. doi: 10.1111/bjd.12557.
7. Deng S, May BH, Zhang AL, Lu C, Xue CC. Topical herbal formulae in the management of psoriasis: systematic review with meta-analysis of

clinical studies and investigation of the pharmacological actions of the main herbs. *Phytother Res* 2014 Apr;**28**(4):480–97. doi: 10.1002/ptr.5028. Epub 2013 Jul 1.

8. Deng S, May BH, Zhang AL, Lu C, Xue CC. Topical herbal medicine combined with pharmacotherapy for psoriasis: a systematic review and meta-analysis. *Arch Dermatol Res* 2013 Apr;**305**(3):179–89. doi: 10.1007/s00403-013-1316-y. Epub 2013 Jan 26.
9. May BH, Zhang AL, Zhou W, Lu CJ, Deng S, Xue CC. Oral herbal medicines for psoriasis: a review of clinical studies. *Chin J Integr Med* 2012 Mar;**18**(3):172–8. doi: 10.1007/s11655-012-1008-z. Epub 2012 Apr 2.
10. May BH, Deng S, Zhang AL, Lu C, Xue CC. In silico database screening of potential targets and pathways of compounds contained in plants used for psoriasis vulgaris. *Arch Dermatol Res* 2015 Jul 5.
11. Zhang CS, Yang L, Zhang AL, May BH, Yu JJ, Guo X, Lu C, Xue CC. Is Oral Chinese Herbal Medicine Beneficial for Psoriasis Vulgaris? A Meta-Analysis of Comparisons with Acitretin. *J Altern Complement Med.* 2016 Mar; 22(3):174–88.
12. Yang L, Zhang CS, May B, Yu J, Guo X, Zhang AL, Xue CC, Lu C. Efficacy of combining oral Chinese herbal medicine and NB-UVB in treating psoriasis vulgaris: a systematic review and meta-analysis. *Chin Med.* 2015 Sep 26; 10:27. doi: 10.1186/s13020-015-0060-y. eCollection 2015.

Authors and Contributors

CO-EDITORS-IN-CHIEF

Prof. Charlie Changli Xue *(RMIT University, Australia)*
Prof. Chuanjian Lu *(Guangdong Provincial Hospital of Chinese Medicine, China)*

CO-DEPUTY EDITORS-IN-CHIEF

Dr. Anthony Lin Zhang *(RMIT University, Australia)*
Dr. Brian H. May *(RMIT University, Australia)*
Prof. Xinfeng Guo *(Guangdong Provincial Hospital of Chinese Medicine, China)*
Prof. Zehuai Wen *(Guangdong Provincial Hospital of Chinese Medicine, China)*

LEAD AUTHORS

Dr. Claire Shuiqing Zhang *(RMIT University, Australia)*
Dr. Jingjie Yu *(Guangdong Provincial Hospital of Chinese Medicine, China)*

CO-AUTHORS

RMIT University (Australia):
Dr. Meaghan Coyle
Dr. Brian H. May
Dr. Anthony Lin Zhang
Prof. Charlie Changli Xue

Guangdong Provincial Hospital of Chinese Medicine (China):

Dr. Yuhong Yan
Dr. Lihong Yang
Dr. Danni Yao
Prof. Xinfeng Guo
Prof. Chuanjian Lu

Members of Advisory Committee and Panel

CO-CHAIRS OF PROJECT PLANNING COMMITTEE

Prof. Peter J Coloe *(RMIT University, Australia)*
Prof. Yubo Lyu *(Guangdong Provincial Hospital of Chinese Medicine, China)*
Prof. Dacan Chen *(Guangdong Provincial Hospital of Chinese Medicine, China)*

CENTRE ADVISORY COMMITTEE (ALPHABETICAL ORDER)

Prof. Keji Chen *(The Chinese Academy of Sciences, China)*
Prof. Aiping Lu *(Hong Kong Baptist University, China)*
Prof. Caroline Smith *(University of Western Sydney, Australia)*
Prof. David F Story *(RMIT University, Australia)*

METHODOLOGY EXPERT ADVISORY PANEL (ALPHABETICAL ORDER)

Prof. Zhaoxiang Bian *(Hong Kong Baptist University, China)*
Prof. George Lewith *(University of Southampton, United Kingdom)*
Prof. Jianping Liu *(Beijing University of Chinese Medicine, China)*
Prof. Frank Thien *(Monash University, Australia)*
Prof. Jialiang Wang *(Sichuan University, China)*

CONTENT EXPERT ADVISORY PANEL

Prof. Yin-ku Lin *(Chang Gung Memorial Hospital at Keelung, Taiwan)*

Prof. Ruiqiang Fan *(Guangdong Provincial Hospital of Chinese Medicine, China)*

Professor Charlie Changli Xue, PhD

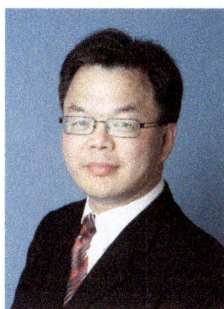

Professor Charlie Changli Xue holds a Bachelor of Medicine (majoring in Chinese Medicine) from Guangzhou University of Chinese Medicine, China (1987) and a PhD from RMIT University, Australia (2000). He has been an academic, researcher, regulator and practitioner for almost three decades. Prof. Xue has made significant contributions to evidence-based educational development, clinical research, regulatory framework and policy development and provision of high quality clinical care to the community. Prof. Xue is recognised internationally as an expert in evidence-based traditional medicine and integrative healthcare.

Prof. Xue is the Inaugural National Chair of the Chinese Medicine Board of Australia appointed by the Australian Health Workforce Ministerial Council (in 2011), and he was reappointed for a second term in 2014. Since 2007, he has been a member of the World Health Organization (WHO) Expert Advisory Panel for Traditional and Complementary Medicine, Geneva. Prof. Xue is also Honorary Senior Principal Research Fellow at the Guangdong Provincial Academy of Chinese Medical Sciences, China.

At RMIT, Prof. Xue is Executive Dean, School of Health and Biomedical Sciences. He is also Director, World Health Organization (WHO) Collaborating Centre for Traditional Medicine.

Between 1995 and 2010, Prof. Xue was Discipline Head of Chinese Medicine at RMIT University. He leads the development of five successful undergraduate and postgraduate degree programs in Chinese Medicine at RMIT University, which is now a global leader in Chinese medicine education and research.

Prof. Xue's research has been supported by over AU$15 million research grants, including six project grants from the Australian Government's National Health & Medical Research Council (NHMRC) and two Australian Research Council (ARC) grants. He has contributed over 200 publications and has been frequently invited as keynote speakers for numerous national and international conferences. Prof. Xue has contributed to over 300 media interviews on issues related to complementary medicine education, research, regulation and practice.

Professor Chuanjian Lu, MD

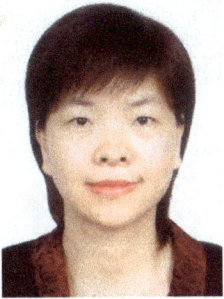

Professor Chuanjian Lu, Doctor of Medicine. She is the vice president of Guangdong Provincial Hospital of Chinese Medicine (Guangdong Provincial Academy of Chinese Medical Sciences, Second Clinical Medical College of Guangzhou University of Chinese Medicine). She also is the chair of the Guangdong Traditional Chinese Medicine (TCM) Standardisation Technical Committee, and the vice-chair of the Immunity Specialty Committee of the World Federation of Chinese Medicine Societies (WFCMS).

Prof. Lu has engaged in scientific research into TCM, clinical practice and teaching for some 25 years. Her research has been devoted to integrated traditional and western medicine. She has edited and published 12 monographs and 120 academic research articles as first author and corresponding author with over 30 articles being included in SCI journals.

She has received widespread recognition for her achievements with awards for "Excellent Teacher of South China," "National Outstanding Women TCM Doctor," and "National Outstanding Young Doctor of TCM." She has also received "The Science and Technology Star of the Association of Chinese Medicine," the "National Excellent Science and Technology Workers of China

Award" and the "Five-Continent Women's Scientific Awards of China Medical Women's Association."

Prof. Lu has won the Award of Science and Technology Progress over 10 times from the Guangdong Provincial Government, the China Association of the Chinese Medicine and the Chinese Hospital Association.

Acknowledgments

The authors and contributors would like to acknowledge the valuable contribution of research assistants and students who assisted with electronic database searching and screening for evaluation of clinical evidence.

Contents

Contents

Contents

List of Figures

List of Tables

1

Introduction to Psoriasis Vulgaris

Overview

Psoriasis vulgaris is a chronic skin condition estimated to affect 2–4% of the population globally. It is characterised by sharply marginated patches of papules and plaques covered with silvery scales, and is often accompanied by itching (pruritus) and pain. Psoriasis often occurs in the teenage years, and is more prevalent in younger females. Psoriasis has a significant impact on quality of life due to physical appearance and time required to treat lesions and maintain clothing and bedding. The economic cost of psoriasis is substantial, including direct costs of management and indirect costs due to loss of productivity. Management in conventional medicine is determined by the severity of the disease, with topical agents used for mild disease and systemic agents used for severe disease. This chapter describes the risk factors for psoriasis, pathological process, diagnosis and severity assessment, and pharmacological and non-pharmacological management.

Psoriasis is a chronic, inflammatory and systemic disease that manifests most commonly as well-circumscribed, erythematous papules and plaques on the skin that are covered with silvery scales. Usually the skin lesions are pruritic and painful with adherent thick scales; removal of these scales may reveal pinpoint bleeding. The disease is a chronic recurring condition that varies in severity from minor localised patches to complete body coverage. Nails and joints can also be affected by psoriasis.[1]

Psoriasis is classified into seven categories: psoriasis vulgaris (plaque psoriasis), guttate psoriasis, inverse psoriasis, nail disease, psoriatic arthritis, pustular psoriasis and erythrodermic psoriasis (Table 1.1).

1

Table 1.1   Types of Psoriasis

Psoriasis Types	Characteristics
Plaque psoriasis (psoriasis vulgaris)	Plaque psoriasis appears as sharply marginated, erythematous patches or plaques with a characteristic silvery-white micaceous scale. The plaques are round or oval in shape and are typically located on the scalp, trunk, buttocks and limbs, especially on extensor surfaces such as the elbows and knees.
Guttate psoriasis	Typical manifestation are dew-drop-like, 1–15-mm, salmon-pink papules, usually with a fine scale. It is found primarily on the trunk and the proximal extremities. The disease is most common during childhood or adolescence and can transition into psoriasis vulgaris.
Inverse psoriasis	Inverse psoriasis commonly appears in the inframammary and abdominal folds, groin, axillae and genitalia. The lesions appear as erythematous plaques with small scales.
Nail disease	The characteristics of nail psoriasis include pitting, onycholysis, subungual hyperkeratosis and the oil-drop sign (a translucent discolouration in the nail bed that resembles a drop of oil beneath the nail plate). It is seen in 90% of patients with psoriatic arthritis.
Psoriatic arthritis	The characteristics of psoriatic arthritis are stiffness, pain, swelling and tenderness of the joints and surrounding ligaments and tendons (dactylitis and enthesitis). The radiographic features of psoriatic arthritis mainly involve joint erosion, joint space narrowing and bony proliferation. Nail damage is very common in psoriatic arthritis.
Pustular psoriasis	Pustular psoriasis consists of (i) generalised pustular psoriasis: shows widespread pustules often on an erythematous background and (ii) localised pustular psoriasis: presents as pustules on the palms of hands and/or soles of the feet.
Erythrodermic psoriasis	Chronic plaque psoriasis may develop into erythrodermic psoriasis. The patient's entire body surface area may be covered with erythema accompanied by varying degrees of scaling, which may lead to hypothermia and dehydration.

Among these seven types, psoriasis vulgaris is the most common type of psoriasis, observed in approximately 80–90% of patients.[1] Psoriasis vulgaris appears as sharply marginated, erythematous patches or plaques with a characteristic silvery-white micaceous scale. The plaques are round or oval in shape and are typically located on the scalp, trunk, buttocks and limbs, especially on extensor surfaces such as the elbows and knees.[1]

The prevalence of psoriasis varies considerably. It is reported that the average global prevalence of psoriasis is approximately 2–4%.[2] The prevalence in cooler regions is higher than that of other regions.[3] It has been suggested that the onset of psoriasis occurs at a younger age in female patients compared with males, which results in a higher prevalence in young females.[4] Furthermore, the mean age of onset for the first presentation of psoriasis is between 15 and 20 years, with a second peak often occurring between 55 and 60 years, and then a significant decline after the age of 70 years, irrespective of gender.[4]

The cost of psoriasis vulgaris is considerable because of its long-term duration. Studies in Germany suggested that the average annual costs of mild psoriasis vulgaris per patient ranged from €500 to €2,000 and for severe disease from €4,000 to €10,000.[5,6] The indirect cost was estimated to be about €1,600 per person per annum.[6] A survey investigating patients with psoriasis in the UK indicated that an average psoriasis patient was absent from work for 26 days a year. In America, psoriasis costs US$11.3 billion in healthcare annually (when calculated at 2% prevalence) and the loss in productivity from psoriasis is around US$16.5 billion per year.[7]

Although psoriasis itself is not a life-threating condition, the physical and psychological comorbidities of psoriasis can significantly impair a patient's quality of life.[8–10] One study compared quality of life in people with psoriasis to people who have other diseases, and found that the decreased quality of life of patients with psoriasis was more severe than that of patients with diabetes, coronary heart disease and cancer.[11] Besides the patient's appearance, the amount of time required to treat extensive skin or scalp lesions and to maintain clothing and bedding adversely affects quality of life as well. In addition, arthritic psoriasis can also result in increasing and debilitating joint pain and stiffness and impaired movement.[12]

Risk Factors

The risk factors of psoriasis are not well defined. However, obesity is believed to be associated with psoriasis because usually patients have a higher body mass index compared with the non-psoriatic population.[13] Smoking is likely to play a role in the onset of psoriasis[14] and alcohol may influence the progression of the disease.[15] Stress is an important trigger factor and may influence the development of the condition.[16] Furthermore, some medications may be associated with the onset or exacerbation of psoriasis, including antimalarial medications, non-steroidal anti-inflammatory drugs (NSAIDs), β-blockers, lithium salts and withdrawal from steroids.[17] Bacterial infections may also trigger or exacerbate psoriasis.[17] Conversely, the consumption of fruit and vegetables, carrots, tomatoes and other food that are rich in β-carotene can decrease the risk of psoriasis.[18]

Pathological Processes

The aetiology and pathogenesis of psoriasis have not been completely defined but immune stimulation of epidermal keratinocytes is involved, where it triggers a complex immunological and inflammatory reaction.[1] Currently, psoriasis is understood as an immune-mediated inflammatory disease in which intra-lesional inflammation primes basal stem keratinocytes to hyper-proliferate and perpetuate the disease process.[1,19,20] The pathogenesis of psoriasis has a large hereditary component. At least eight chromosomal loci have been identified for which statistically significant evidence for linkage to psoriasis has been observed.[1] In addition, environmental factors including infection, smoking, medications (e.g. β-blockers, NSAIDs, antimalarials, terbinafine, calcium channel blockers, lipid-lowering drugs), skin injury (Koebner's phenomenon) and stress are thought to evoke an inflammatory response and subsequent hyper-proliferation of keratinocytes, resulting in psoriasis.[1,19]

Diagnosis

Symptom Assessment

The diagnosis of psoriasis vulgaris is based on typical lesion morphology and clinical history.[19,21] The Auspitz sign (bleeding that occurs after psoriasis scales have been removed) is regarded as the key to diagnosing psoriasis, comprising (i) plaques covered by silvery-white scales which shows the typical candle wax phenomenon after scratching; (ii) punctate bleeding when the covering skin is removed and (iii) pinpoint bleeding.[19] Identifying the time of onset of lesions, possible triggers, related symptoms (i.e. itch, pain, sensitivity, irritation) and family history are essential to informing the diagnosis.[21] In some cases, histological examination of biopsies taken from the border of representative lesions is needed to confirm the diagnosis.[19,22]

Evaluation of Psoriasis Symptom Severity

To some extent, evaluating the severity is more complicated than diagnosing psoriasis. Clinically, dermatologists often combine objective evaluation of lesion location, thickness, symptoms, presence or absence of psoriatic arthritis with the subjective assessment of the physical, financial and emotional impact of the disease on the patient's quality of life to determine the disease severity.[1] Various outcome measures are used to evaluate psoriasis symptom severity. The Psoriasis Area and Severity Index (PASI), PGA, Body Surface Area (BSA) and the Dermatology Life Quality Index (DLQI) are most commonly used.[1,19] The PASI is a tool to assess the overall psoriasis severity based on lesion area, erythema, induration and scaling.[23] It is a non-linear measure (range 0–72) and scores of ten or more have been shown to correlate with a number of indicators of severe disease.[22] However, the PASI score is not sensitive to change when body surface area <10%, and has not been validated in children where assessments for BSA may be inaccurate.[22] The DLQI is used primarily to determine Health-Related Quality of Life (HRQoL).[24] The combination of PASI and DLQI are applied to evaluate the effectiveness of treatment.[19] PGA is an average assessment of all psoriatic lesions, regardless of quantifying BSA or evaluating individual lesion locations.[25]

For the classification of disease severity, there is no widely accepted definition of what represents mild, moderate or severe psoriasis, but the following criteria outlines how the disease often is classified in practice:[26]

- Mild to moderate psoriasis: Good control of lesions with topical therapies alone; <10% of body affected
- Moderate psoriasis: Topical therapy still able to control the disease; >10% of body affected
- Moderate to severe psoriasis: Topical therapies fail to control the disease; >10% of body affected. Very thick lesions located in 'difficult-to-treat' regions, such as the palms and soles
- Severe psoriasis: Systemic treatments are required to control the disease; >20% of body affected. Very intense local signs with very thick lesions and >10% of body affected may also be considered as severe.

Differential Diagnosis

The clinical diagnosis of psoriasis is relatively easy, especially when the lesions consist of erythematous, silvery-white scales and indurated plaques that are sharply demarcated and distributed symmetrically on the extensor surfaces of limbs, the lower back and the scalp. Differential diagnosis of plaque psoriasis (psoriasis vulgaris) should focus on nummular eczema tinea, mycosis fungoides and pityriasis rosea. Predilection sites and the nails' appearance may aid diagnosis. Sometimes a skin biopsy may be useful to confirm the diagnosis.[1]

Management

For the management of psoriasis vulgaris, many treatment options exist. Topical medications are typically used for mild disease, phototherapy for moderate disease and systemic agents for severe disease.

Commonly used topical medications include calcineurin inhibitors, dithranol/anthralin, corticosteroids, coal tar, Tazarotene, vitamin D3 and vitamin D3-analogues, salicylic acid and non-medicated topical moisturizers.[19] Phototherapy and photochemotherapy are effective for the management of psoriasis vulgaris. Phototherapy involves UVA and UVB wavelengths. Originally, broadband UVB light was used for psoriasis treatment. Narrowband UVB (NB-UVB) later became possible after the development of fluorescent narrowband UVB tubes. Photochemotherapy, the administration of psoralens (photosensitising agents found in plants) followed by UVA phototherapy (PUVA), has been shown to be effective for clearing psoriasis.[19,27] Commonly used systemic medications include retinoids (vitamin A derivatives), methotrexate, cyclosporine and fumaric acid esters. Systemic treatment, alone or in combination with topical treatment are usually used for severe psoriasis vulgaris cases. Biologics such as TNF inhibitors and T-cell inhibitors are also used in the treatment of psoriasis vulgaris.[19]

Although pharmacological therapy and phototherapy have been shown to be effective, they often are associated with side effects. For example, most topical agents may cause localised skin irritation including burning, pruritus, oedema, peeling, dryness and erythema; oral retinoids (acitretin) have been associated with birth defects and liver damage; oral methotrexate may cause liver toxicity; NB-UVB phototherapy is associated with itching and blistering of the treated skin, irritation of the eyes or cold sores; and PUVA is associated with nausea, headache, fatigue, burning and itching. Biologics have been associated with a small increase in the risk of infection, and clinical guidelines regard biologics as third-line treatment for psoriasis vulgaris following inadequate response to topical treatment, phototherapy, and non-biologic systemic treatments.[19]

Furthermore, climatotherapy can also be used as psoriasis vulgaris treatment. Climatotherapy consists of staying for long periods of time in geographical regions with a large amount of sunlight, with schemes usually varying by institution/treatment site.[19] Given the considerable psychosocial burden of psoriasis, educational programmes are an important and economical form of additional psychosocial treatment of the disease. Psychosocial therapy can be offered as an adjunct to

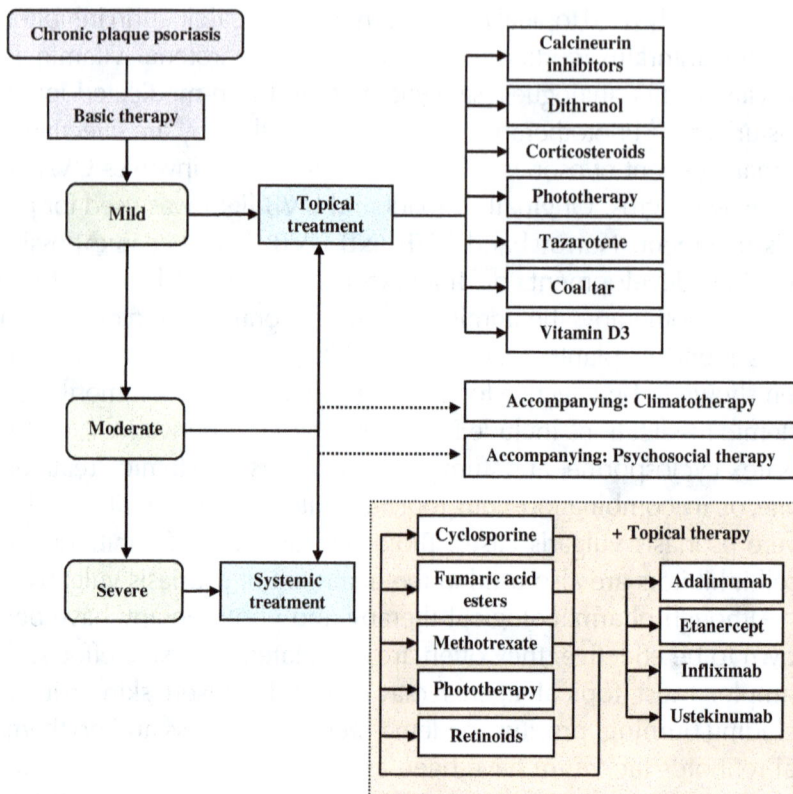

Figure 1.1 Overview of evaluated therapy options for use in chronic psoriasis vulgaris (adapted from S3-Guidelines on the Treatment of Psoriasis Vulgaris).

topical or systemic treatments. Clinical experience suggests that psychosocial therapy tends to benefit patients with chronic recurrent disease more than those with chronic stable psoriasis.[19]

Treatment Goals

When treating psoriasis vulgaris, the complete absence of cutaneous symptoms is not achievable in all patients. In recent years, clinical studies have used PASI 75 (a 75% reduction of PASI score) as the goal of psoriasis therapies. In most studies, the expected treatment duration for achieving PASI 75 is 10–16 weeks. Therefore, PASI 75 has been set as the treatment goal by current clinical guidelines. Furthermore, the 'lower hurdle' (minimum target) of PASI 50 (a 50% reduction of PASI score) was also established. With regard to quality of life, the goal of psoriasis therapy is to achieve a DLQI score of 0 or 1, meaning that the patient no longer experiences any impairment of quality of life due to skin symptoms. A DLQI score of less than five can be taken as the minimum treatment target. If this minimum target is not reached within a given amount of time, the therapy must be modified. For example, for fast-acting drugs (e.g. infliximab), treatment goals should be set at ten weeks for induction therapy, while for slower-acting drugs (e.g. fumaric acid esters, MTX), the expected treatment duration should be 16 weeks.[19]

An overview of evaluated treatment options for chronic psoriasis vulgaris is shown in Figure 1.1.

A summary of this chapter can be seen in Table 1.2.

Table 1.2   Chapter Summary of Psoriasis Vulgaris in Conventional Medicine

Definition of psoriasis	• Chronic, inflammatory and systemic disease • Well-circumscribed, erythematous papules and plaques covered with silvery scales • Nails and joints can also be affected by psoriasis
Classification of psoriasis	• Psoriasis vulgaris (plaque psoriasis) • Inverse psoriasis • Erythrodermic psoriasis • Pustular psoriasis • Guttate psoriasis • Nail disease • Psoriatic arthritis
Diagnosis of psoriasis	• Based on clinical evaluation of the skin lesions • X-ray assist the diagnosis of psoriatic arthritis
Management of psoriasis	• Topical therapies (calcineurin inhibitors, dithranol/anthralin, corticosteriods, coal tar, tazarotene, vitamin D3 and vitamin D3-analogues, salicylic acid) • Systemic treatments (cyclosporine, fumaric acid esters, methotrexate, retinoids, etc.) • Biologics • Other therapies (phototherapy and photochemotherapy, climatotherapy, education programmes and psychosocial therapy)

References

1. Menter A, Gottlieb A, Feldman SR, van Voorhees AS, Leonardi CL, Gordon KB, *et al.* (2008) Guidelines of care for the management of psoriasis and psoriatic arthritis: Section 1. Overview of psoriasis and guidelines of care for the treatment of psoriasis with biologics. *J Am Acad Dermatol* **58**(5): 826–850.
2. Enamandram M, Kimball AB. (2013) Psoriasis epidemiology: The interplay of genes and the environment. *J Invest Dermatol* **133**(2): 287–289.
3. Neimann AL, Shin DB, Wang X, Margolis DJ, Troxel AB, Gelfand JM. (2006) Prevalence of cardiovascular risk factors in patients with psoriasis. *J Am Acad Dermatol* **55**(5): 829–835.
4. Gelfand JM, Weinstein R, Porter SB, Neimann AL, Berlin JA, Margolis DJ. (2005) Prevalence and treatment of psoriasis in the United Kingdom: A population-based study. *Arch Dermatol* **141**(12): 1537–1541.
5. Berger K, Ehlken B, Kugland B, Augustin M. (2005) Cost-of-illness in patients with moderate and severe chronic psoriasis vulgaris in Germany. *J Dtsch Dermatol Ges* **3**(7): 511–518.
6. Schoffski O, Augustin M, Prinz J, Rauner K, Schubert E, Sohn S, *et al.* (2007) Costs and quality of life in patients with moderate to severe plaque-type psoriasis in Germany: A multi-center study. *J Dtsch Dermatol Ges* **5**(3): 209–218.
7. Beyer V, Wolverton SE. (2010) Recent trends in systemic psoriasis treatment costs. *Arch Dermatol* **146**(1): 46–54.
8. Krueger G, Koo J, Lebwohl M, Menter A, Stern RS, Rolstad T. (2001) The impact of psoriasis on quality of life: Results of a 1998 National Psoriasis Foundation patient-membership survey. *Arch Dermatol* **137**(3): 280–284.
9. Russo PA, Ilchef R, Cooper AJ. (2004) Psychiatric morbidity in psoriasis: A review. *Aust J Dermatol* **45**(3): 155–159.
10. Sampogna F, Tabolli S, Abeni D. (2012) Living with psoriasis: Prevalence of shame, anger, worry, and problems in daily activities and social life. *Acta Dermatol Venereol* **92**(3): 299–303.
11. Rapp SR, Feldman SR, Exum ML, Fleischer AB, Jr., Reboussin DM. (1999) Psoriasis causes as much disability as other major medical diseases. *J Am Acad Dermatol* **41**(3 Pt. 1): 401–407.
12. Clarke P. (2011) Psoriasis. *Aust Fam Phys* **40**(7): 468–473.
13. Setty AR, Curhan G, Choi HK. (2007) Obesity, waist circumference, weight change, and the risk of psoriasis in women: Nurses' Health Study II. *Arch Intern Med* **167**(15): 1670–1675.

14. Herron MD, Hinckley M, Hoffman MS, Papenfuss J, Hansen CB, Callis KP, *et al.* (2005) Impact of obesity and smoking on psoriasis presentation and management. *Arch Dermatol* **141**(12): 1527–1534.
15. Higgins E. (2000) Alcohol, smoking and psoriasis. *Clin Exp Dermatol* **25**(2): 107–110.
16. Naldi L, Chatenoud L, Linder D, Belloni Fortina A, Peserico A, Virgili AR, *et al.* (2005) Cigarette smoking, body mass index, and stressful life events as risk factors for psoriasis: Results from an Italian case-control study. *J Invest Dermatol* **125**(1): 61–67.
17. Perera GK, di Meglio P, Nestle FO. Psoriasis. (2012) *Annu Rev Pathol* **7**: 385–422.
18. Naldi L, Parazzini F, Peli L, Chatenoud L, Cainelli T. (1996) Dietary factors and the risk of psoriasis: Results of an Italian case-control study. *Br J Dermatol* **134**(1): 101–106.
19. Nast A, Boehncke WH, Mrowietz U, Ockenfels HM, Philipp S, Reich K, *et al.* (2012) S3 — Guidelines on the treatment of psoriasis vulgaris (English version). Update. *J Dtsch Dermatol Ges* **10** (Suppl. 2): S1–S95.
20. Nestle FO, Kaplan DH, Barker J. (2009) Psoriasis. *N Engl J Med* **361**(5): 496–509.
21. Gottlieb A, Korman NJ, Gordon KB, Feldman SR, Lebwohl M, Koo JY, *et al.* (2008) Guidelines of care for the management of psoriasis and psoriatic arthritis: Section 2. Psoriatic arthritis: Overview and guidelines of care for treatment with an emphasis on the biologics. *J Am Acad Dermatol* **58**(5): 851–864.
22. National Clinical Guideline Centre. (2012) Psoriasis assessment and management of psoriasis. Retrieved from https://www.nice.org.uk/guidance/cg153
23. Marks R, Barton SP, Shuttleworth D, Finlay AY. (1989) Assessment of disease progress in psoriasis. *Arch Dermatol* **125**(2): 235–240.
24. Finlay AY, Khan GK. (1994) Dermatology Life Quality Index (DLQI) — A simple practical measure for routine clinical use. *Clin Exp Dermatol* **19**(3): 210–216.
25. Robinson A, Kardos M, Kimball AB. (2012) Physician Global Assessment (PGA) and Psoriasis Area and Severity Index (PASI): Why do both? A systematic analysis of randomized controlled trials of biologic agents for moderate to severe plaque psoriasis. *J Am Acad Dermatol* **66**(3): 369–375.
26. Therapeutic Goods Administration, Department of Health. (2004) Guideline on clinical investigation of medicinal products indicated

for the treatment of psoriasis. Retrieved from https://www.tga.gov.au/clinical-efficacy-and-safety-guidelines

27. Menter A, Korman NJ, Elmets CA, Feldman SR, Gelfand JM, Gordon KB, *et al.* (2010) Guidelines of care for the management of psoriasis and psoriatic arthritis: Section 5. Guidelines of care for the treatment of psoriasis with phototherapy and photochemotherapy. *J Am Acad Dermatol* **62**(1): 114–135.

2

Psoriasis Vulgaris in Chinese Medicine

Overview

In Chinese medicine (CM), psoriasis vulgaris is considered to develop as a result of failure of the nourishing and cooling functions of Blood. Causes include emotional disturbance leading to *qi* stagnation and then Blood heat, external or internal wind leading to dryness, and long-term heat in the Blood leading to Blood stasis. Syndrome differentiation is used to guide treatment, with various options including Chinese herbal medicine and acupuncture therapies. This chapter describes the key Chinese medicine syndromes seen in psoriasis vulgaris. Treatments are described based on key clinical texts and practice guidelines, and include Chinese herbal medicine (CHM), acupuncture and related therapies, and dietary and lifestyle advice.

The Chinese term '*Bai bi*' (白疕) is the most likely of all classical terms to correspond with the modern understanding of psoriasis.[1,2] Despite diversity in the understanding of the pathogenesis of psoriasis, the fundamental pathogenesis is attributed to Blood syndromes. Blood originates from the (i) food *qi* produced by the Spleen. Through the descending of (ii) Lung *qi* (气), the (iii) food *qi* is sent to the Heart, and is then transformed into Blood. Blood has the function of nourishing and moistening. Besides the nourishing action of *qi*, Blood can moisten the skin and hair, which ensures the tissues are not too dry.[3] Multiple pathogenic factors may cause Blood heat, Blood deficiency or Blood stasis, which will impact on the function of Blood.

Aetiology and Pathogenesis

Blood heat can be caused by multiple factors. For instance, depression and long-term emotional disturbance causes stasis of *qi* which can turn to heat and result in Heart fire. Overindulgence in fish, seafood or meat may lead to disharmony between the Spleen and Stomach, resulting in stagnation of *qi*, which can transform into heat.[4,5] For people with a constitutional predisposition to Blood heat syndromes, the coupling of Blood heat syndrome with an external invasion of wind can cause internal wind leading to dryness. Wind-dryness will exhaust the body fluids and Blood, and further result in deficiency of the *yin* (阴) and Blood dryness. Therefore, the lack of nourishment from body fluids and Blood will lead to the psoriasis symptoms of dry skin and scaly skin.[6] Heat in the nutrient Blood can scorch the Blood and result in Blood stasis. Long-term Blood stasis may transform into heat and exacerbate Blood heat. Blood stasis is an important factor when the disease is complicated and/or of prolonged duration.[1,7,8]

Syndromes Differentiation and Treatments

Syndrome differentiation is an important feature of diagnosis in CM dermatology. The *Standard of Diagnosis and Assessment of Treatment Effects of Dermatological Conditions in Chinese Medicine* published in 1994 by the State Administration of Traditional Chinese Medicine of the People's Republic of China states that the main syndrome types of *Bai bi* (psoriasis) are 'wind-heat and Blood dryness', 'Blood deficiency and wind-dryness' and 'Blood stasis in the skin'.[2] The *Evidence-Based Guidelines of Clinical Practice in Chinese Medicine* published by the Chinese Academy of Chinese Medical Sciences in 2011 also describes the same syndromes. In detailing the treatment principles for these syndromes, slightly different terminologies were used (Blood heat, Blood dryness and Blood stasis); however, the clinical presentations are consistent with the described syndromes.[1] Findings from a review of syndromes included in reports of expert experience, case-control studies and randomised controlled trials (RCTs) from 1979–2010, indicated that Blood heat, Blood dryness and Blood stasis are the basic syndrome types.[9]

Therefore, the treatment principle of psoriasis vulgaris mainly targets the Blood.

The following guidelines on the diagnosis and treatment of psoriasis vulgaris were used as references in the following section. They include the *Standard of Diagnosis and Assessment of Treatment Effects of Dermatological Conditions in Chinese Medicine* published in 1994 by the State Administration of Traditional Chinese Medicine of the People's Republic of China,[2] *Evidence-Based Guidelines of Clinical Practice in Chinese Medicine* published by the Chinese Academy of Chinese Medicinal Sciences[1] and the *Guidelines for Diagnosis and Treatment of Common Diseases of Dermatology in Traditional Chinese Medicine.*[12]

Oral CHM Treatment Based on Syndrome Differentiation

Blood Heat

Clinical manifestations: new bright red papules or maculopapules of varying sizes develop continuously, Auspitz's sign when the scale is removed, Koebner's phenomenon occurs occasionally. Accompanying symptoms include itching, anxiety, dry mouth, constipation and yellow urine; red tongue with yellow or greasy coating. The pulse is slippery, string or rapid.[1,2,10,11]

Treatment principle: Clear heat and cool the Blood, relieve toxicity and reduce erythema[10,11]

Formula: Modified *Xiao feng san* plus *Xi jiao di huang tang,*[10,11] modified *Liang xue di huang tang.*[12]

Herbs: *Dang gui, sheng di huang, fang feng, chan tui, zhi mu, ku shen, hu ma ren, jing jie, cang zhu, niu bang zi, shi gao, shui niu jiao, chi shao, mu dan pi.*

Analysis of formula: *Sheng di huang, shui niu jiao, chi shao* and *mu dan pi* clear heat, cool the Blood and relieve toxicity. *Dang gui* and *hu ma ren* nourish the Blood and moisten dryness. *Jing jie, fang feng, niu bang zi* and *chan tui* disperse external wind to stop itch. *Cang zhu* and *ku shen* clear damp-heat. *Shi gao* and *zhi mu* clears *qi* level heat.

Manufactured medicines: *Fu fang qing dai wan* (pill),[1,13] which can clear heat and relieve toxicity, remove Blood stasis and reduce erythema.

Blood Dryness

Clinical manifestations: Long-term disease, lesions manifest as light red and patchy, covered with plenty of dry silvery-white scales. Parts of lesions have disappeared. Dry and chapped skin with itch or pain. Accompanying symptoms include dry mouth, constipation; red tongue body with a thin and white coating. The pulse is wiry and slow.[1,2,10,11]

Treatment principle: Tonify *yin* and nourish the Blood, moisten dryness and dispel wind.[10,11]

Formula: Modified *Dang gui yin zi*,[10,12] *Yang xue run fu yin*.[12]

Herbs: *Dang gui, sheng di huang, bai shao, chuan xiong, he shou wu, jing jie, fang feng, bai ji li, huang qi, sheng gan cao, tian dong, mai dong, tian hua fen*.

Analysis of formula: *Dang gui, he shou wu* and *huang qi* nourish the Blood and moisten dryness. *Sheng di huang, bai shao* and *chuan xiong* clear heat, cool and invigorate the Blood. *Jing jie, fang feng* and *bai ji li* dispel wind. *Tian dong, mai dong* and *tian hua fen* tonify *yin* and moisten dryness. *Sheng gan cao* clears heat and harmonizes the actions of the other herbs.

Manufactured medicines: *Xiao yin ke li* (granule),[1] which can clear heat and cool the Blood, nourish the Blood and moisten dryness, dispel wind and stop pruritus.

Blood Stasis

Clinical manifestations: The disease duration is long and at the stable stage. Dull red, hard and thick plaques are covered by thick, dry, silvery-white scales, with itch. There are no obvious general symptoms but there is a dark purple or red tongue body with petechial spots. The pulse is uneven, or wiry and slow.[1,2,10,11]

Treatment principle: Invigorate the Blood and transform Blood stasis, nourish the Blood and moisten dryness.[10,11,13]

Formula: Modified *Tao hong si wu tang*.[10,11,13]

Herbs: *Shu di huang, dang gui, bai shao, chuan xiong, tao ren, hong hua*.

Analysis of formula: *Shu di huang* tonifies the *yin* and nourishes the Blood. *Bai shao* tonifies the Liver Blood and preserves the *yin*. *Dang gui* tonifies the Blood and nourishes the Liver. *Chuan xiong* invigorates the Blood and promotes the movement of *qi*. *Tao ren* and *hong hua* have a very strong effect on invigorating the Blood and transforming Blood stasis.

Manufactured medicines: *Lei gong teng duo gan pian* (tablets),[13] which can dispel wind and relieve toxicity.

Topical Therapies of CHM

In external CHM, psoriasis can be treated with topical preparations such as baths, steaming therapy, enemas and other methods. Among these, CHM ointments and CHM baths are the most commonly used therapies.[1]

CHM Ointment

Mild ointment or moisturizer could be used at the progressive stage,[10,11,13] such as *Huang bo* ointment, *Qing dai* ointment, *Qing dai ma you*,[11,13] *Shi du* ointment, *Pu lian* ointment, *Bing huang fu le* ointment[1] and 10% sulphur ointment could be used for stable and regressive stage.[11,13]

CHM Baths

The herbs used for CHM baths are usually based on syndrome differentiation. Herbs commonly used in CHM bath decoctions are: *xu chang qing, qian li guang, di fu zi, huang bo, she chuang zi, cang er zi, lang du, bai xian pi, tu jin pi,* and/or *huai hua.*[11]

Acupuncture Therapies and Other CM Therapies

Acupuncture including body and auricular acupuncture has been recommended to treat psoriasis. Care must be taken when new lesions are developing, where skin penetration may be more likely to result in Koebner's phenomenon. (see Table 2.1).

Other Management Strategies

Infection and trauma should be avoided, especially upper respiratory tract infections in the period of seasonal change.[1,10,11]

Table 2.1 Summary of Acupuncture and Other CM Therapies for Psoriasis

Intervention	Acupuncture Points/Body Area	Treatment Frequency
Body acupuncture[10,13]	Main points: LI11 *Quchi*, LI4 *Hegu*, GV14 *Dazhui*, BL13 *Feishu*, SP10 *Xuehai*, SP6 *Sanyinjiao*; supplementary points for lesions on the head and face: LI20 *Yingxiang*, GB20 *Fengchi*, SI18 *Quanliao*; supplementary points for lesions on upper limbs: TE6 *Zhigou* for the upper limbs; supplementary points for lesions on lower limbs: ST36 *Zusanli*, ST40 *Fenglong* for the lower limbs	Treatment is applied once a day with ten times as one treatment course
Auricular acupuncture[10,13]	CO14 *Fei*, TF4 *Shenmen*, CO18 *Neifenmi*, CO15 *Xin*, CO7 *Dachang* etc.	Every other day, with ten days as one treatment course

Table 2.2   Summary of Psoriasis Vulgaris in Chinese Medicine

	Blood Heat	**Blood Dryness**	**Blood Stasis**
Oral CHM	Modified *Xiao feng san* plus *Xi jiao di huang tang*, modified *Liang xue di huang tang*	*Dang gui yin zi, Yang xue run fu yin*	Modified *Tao hong si wu tang*
Topical CHM	**CHM ointment**: for progressive stage: *Huang bo* ointment, *Qing dai* ointment, *Qing dai ma you*, *Shi du* ointment, *Pu lian* ointment, *Bing huang fu le* ointment; for stable and regressive stage: 10% sulphur ointment. **CHM baths**: *xu chang qing, qian li guang, di fu zi, huang bo, she chuang zi, cang er zi, lang du, bai xian pi, tu jin pi* and/or *huai hua*		
Acupuncture	Main points: LI11 *Quchi*, LI4 *Hegu*, GV14 *Dazhui*, BL13 *Feishu*, SP10 *Xuehai*, SP6 *Sanyinjiao*		

The diet should avoid spicy food, seafood, beef or mutton. The diet should include considerable amounts of fresh vegetables and fruits. Avoid alcohol and tobacco consumption.[1,10,11]

Regular daily routine, avoid hyper-stress and overwork.

Avoid using high irritation medications topically, especially for acute psoriasis. Do not take baths with very hot water.

A summary of this chapter can be seen in Table 2.2.

References

1. Chinese Academy of Chinese Medical Sciences. (2011) *Evidence-Based Guidelines of Clinical Practice in Chinese Medicine* [in Chinese 中医循证临床实践指南]. Chinese Academy of Chinese Medical Sciences Publishing House, Beijing, People's Republic of China.
2. State Administration of Traditional Chinese Medicine of the People's Republic of China. (1994) *Standard of Diagnosis and Assessment of Treatment Effects of Dermatological Conditions in Chinese Medicine* [in Chinese: 中医病证诊断疗效标准]. Nanjing University Press, Nanjing, People's Republic of China.
3. Maciocia G. (1989) *The Foundations of Chinese Medicine*. Churchill Livingston, Elsevier.

4. Beijing Hospital of TCM. (2006) *Zhao Bing Nan Clinical Volume* [in Chinese: 赵炳南临床经验集]. People's Medical Publishing House, Beijing, People's Republic of China.

5. Chinese Academy of Chinese Medical Sciences. (2001) *Zhang Zhi Li Clinical Dermatology Studies* [in Chinese: 张志礼皮肤病临床经验辑要]. Chinese Academy of Chinese Medical Sciences Publishing House, Beijing, People's Republic of China.

6. Research Institute of Traditional Chinese Medicine of the People's Republic of China, Guang'anmen Hospital. (2005) *Zhu Ren Kang Clinical Volume: Dermatology* [in Chinese: 朱仁康临床经验集]. People's Medical Publishing House, Beijing, People's Republic of China.

7. Yan YH, Lu CJ, Xuan GW. (2012) Exploring the pathogenesis of psoriasis [in Chinese: 寻常型银屑病核心病机探讨]. *Liaoning J Tradit Chin Med* **39**(6): 1013–1015.

8. Wu YJ. (2009) 中医治疗银屑病相关文献的用药规律研究 [in Chinese]. Thesis. Xinjiang Medical University, Xinjiang, People's Republic of China.

9. Lu CJ, Zeng Z, Xie XL, Ning J. (2012) 1979–2010 1979-2010 年寻常型银屑病文献证候分布情况分析 [in Chinese]. *J Tradit Chin Med* **53**(11): 959–961.

10. Li YQ. (2012) 中医外科学 [in Chinese]. Chinese Press of Traditional Chinese Medicine, Beijing, People's Republic of China.

11. Yang 2B, Fan RQ, Dens BX. (2010) 中医皮肤性病学 [in Chinese]. Chinese Press of Traditional Chinese Medicine, Beijing, People's Republic of China.

12. China Association of Chinese Medicine. (2012) 中医皮肤科常见病诊疗指南 [in Chinese]. Chinese Press of Traditional Chinese Medicine, Beijing, People's Republic of China.

13. Chen DC. (2008 中西医结合皮肤性病学 [in Chinese]. Science Press, Beijing, People's Republic of China.

3

Classical Chinese Medicine Literature

Overview

Classical Chinese medicine literature provides a rich source of information for the prevention and management of disease. Many treatments used in contemporary practice date back to classical literature, including current treatments for psoriasis. The Chinese term for psoriasis was standardised in 1956, and prior to this the term, *Bai bi* was used in classical Chinese medicine texts. This chapter describes the findings of a systematic search of the *Zhong Hua Yi Dian*, one of the largest collections of classical Chinese medicine texts available. A selection of search terms was identified from classical dictionaries and texts. A search of the *Zhong Hua Yi Dian* located over 600 citations, which were analysed to identify the common formulae, herbs and acupuncture points used to treat symptoms of psoriasis.

Chinese medicine (CM) therapies have been clinically practised for thousands of years. For example, acupuncture is generally thought to originate in ancient China some 2,500 years ago,[1,2] and the literature on Chinese herbal medicine (CHM) dates back to the oldest surviving book on materia medica, '*Shen Nong Ben Cao Jing*' (Shennong's Materia Medica) which is believed to have originated in the Western Han dynasty (206 BC–24 AD).[3,4] During the thousands of years of CM clinical practice, a voluminous literature has been accumulated, which records descriptions of many skin diseases and treatments. Some of this information has contributed to the development of the contemporary CM clinical management of psoriasis vulgaris. Considering that psoriasis vulgaris is a modern concept, in order to explore the evidence of CM therapies for psoriasis vulgaris management in history, it is important to systematically analyse references to skin disorders in classical CM literature and discuss how the psoriasis-like condition was conceptualised and managed over time. Although classical CM literature is vast, the advent of digitalised collections of the classical CM literature makes it possible to systematically search for such information that could further inform contemporary practice.[3,4]

In China, modern terminology of psoriasis vulgaris was not standardised until the action of the Chinese National Congress of Dermatology in 1956.[5] In this congress, the term *Yin xie bing* (银屑病) was created in the Chinese language to be used for psoriasis vulgaris, replacing the classical term *Bai bi* (白疕) which had been used in classical literature. *Yin* refers to the silvery-white colour of the lesion, *Xie* refers to fragmentary scale and *Bing* means disease. This new term represents the main feature of psoriasis vulgaris — white-coloured scales. *Yin xie bing* had never been used in CM classical literature. However, whether *Bai bi* was a unique term in history or there are other similar classical terms referring to psoriasis vulgaris is uncertain. Some Chinese language CM works (including textbooks, monographs and journal articles) suggested that throughout the history of CM, it is likely that a variety of terms have been used to refer to disorders that corresponded to psoriasis vulgaris as it is now defined.[6,7]

Classical Literature Search

Thirty-three CM works on dermatological conditions were manually searched to identify relevant terms. Fourteen terms were identified: *Bai bi* (白疕), *Gan xuan* (干癣), *Xong pi xuan* (松皮癣), *She shi* (蛇虱), *Bi feng* (疕风), *Bai ke chuang* (白壳疮), *Feng xuan* (风癣), *Gou pi xuan* (狗皮癣), *She feng* (蛇风), *Niu pi xuan* (牛皮癣), *Bai xuan* (白癣), *Yin qian feng* (银钱疯), *Gou xuan* (狗癣) and *She ling chuang* (摄领疮). Among these 14 terms, *She ling chuang* was classified as a neurodermatitis-type condition after consultation with clinical experts, because it 'usually appears in the nape area, itchy and painful, and it is caused/aggravated by the collar of clothing frequently touching or rubbing the skin'. The other 13 terms are classified as possibly related to psoriasis vulgaris to some extent (Table 3.1).

A total of 608 citations were found by searching *Zhong Hua Yi Dian* (ZHYD) with the 13 terms (Figure 3.1). They were derived from 162 different books with the largest proportions of books (41.4%) and citations (50.2%) originating in the Ming dynasty (1368–1644 AD). The book *Pu Ji Fang* (*Prescriptions for Universal Relief*) (1406 AD) produced the highest yield, providing 7.4% (*n* = 45) of all citations. The earliest book was *Zhou Hou Bei Ji Fang* (*Handbook of Prescriptions for Emergencies*) (363 AD), while the most recent one was *Wai Ke Shi San Fang Kao* (*Investigation of Thirteen Formulas for External Medicine*) (1947 AD).

Table 3.1 Terms Used to Identify Classical Literature Citations

Pinyin	Chinese Characters
Bai bi	白疕
Bai ke chuang	白壳疮
Bai xuan	白癣
Bi feng	疕风
Feng xuan	风癣
Gan xuan	干癣
Gou xuan	狗癣
Gou pi xuan	狗皮癣
Niu pi xuan	牛皮癣
She feng	蛇风
She shi	蛇虱
Song pi xuan	松皮癣
Yin qian feng	银钱疯

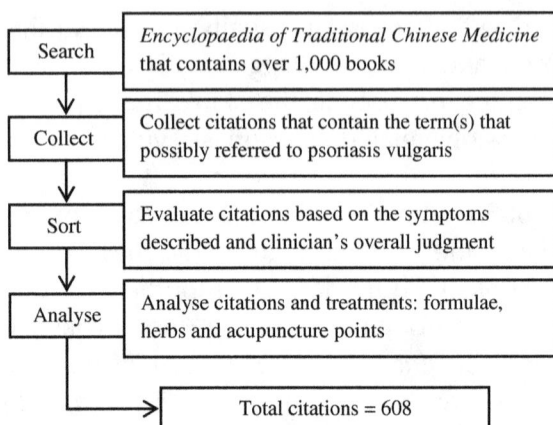

Figure 3.1 Classical literature citations.

The terms of 608 citations were distributed across historical periods. *Gan xuan, Bai xuan, Feng xuan* and *Gou xuan* were the terms that appeared the earliest, before the Tang dynasty (before 618 AD). *Gou xuan* continued into the Qing dynasty while *Gan xuan, Bai xuan* and *Feng xuan* still surfaced in the Minguo period (1912–1949 AD). *Niu pi xuan* appeared in books from the Song/Jin dynasty (960–1271 AD) until the Minguo period. Seven terms (*Bai bi, She shi, Gou pi xuan, Bai ke chuang, She feng, Bi feng* and *Xong pi xuan*) first emerged in the Ming dynasty, and one term, *Yin qian feng*, was used only in the Qing dynasty (1644–1911 AD).

Among the 608 citations, 584 (96.1%) mentioned some sort of skin lesion, 206 (33.9%) stated that itch was a symptom, 165 (27.1%) referred to scaly skin, 101 (16.6%) cited white-coloured skin, 24 (3.9%) mentioned red-coloured skin and 77 (12.7%) stated dry skin. Very few citations specified the absence of a symptom. For the clinicians' overall judgment based on reading the full citation, 84 citations (13.8%) were judged as 'most likely psoriasis vulgaris'. Combining the symptoms described by the citation and clinician's judgment, 60 citations containing 'skin lesion' as well as 'white-coloured skin' were judged as 'most likely psoriasis vulgaris'. These 60 citations were considered as the most likely psoriasis vulgaris citations, and were used for further analysis.

Terms of the Most Likely Psoriasis Vulgaris Citations

Eight terms were used in these 60 citations, as follows: *Bai bi* (*n* = 29), *Gan xuan* (*n* = 28), *She shi* (*n* = 16), *Feng xuan* (*n* = 9), *She feng* (*n* = 2), *Bi feng* (*n* = 2), *Bai ke chuang* (*n* = 1) and *Bai xuan* (*n* = 1). In the case of *Bai bi*, all 29 citations were included in the 60 most likely citations, so it was the term that was most frequently and consistently used for conditions likely to have been psoriasis vulgaris. Similarly, 100% of citations for *She shi* and *Bi feng* were included in this pool. These three terms all first appeared in the Ming dynasty. No other terms were exclusively included in this list.

For the other terms, a 'not psoriasis' judgment was made for 50% of *She feng*, 37% of *Gan xuan*, 17.3% of *Feng xuan*, 16.7% of *Bai ke chuang*, 8% of *Bai xuan* and 6% of *Gou xuan* citations. *Feng xuan* was used in the largest number of citations (*n* = 301), but only six citations (2%) were included in the most likely psoriasis vulgaris pool.

Therefore, *Bai bi*, *She shi* and *Bi feng* are the terms most consistently used to refer to psoriasis vulgaris. They first appeared in the Ming dynasty and *Bai bi* still remains in use. Citations with other terms may have referred to psoriasis vulgaris, but in other cases, these terms could be used for disorders whose descriptions were inconsistent with psoriasis.

Representative Citations

The most representative citation, stating both *Bai bi* and *She shi*, was in the Ming dynasty book *Zheng Zhi Zhun Sheng* (*Standard of Pattern/Syndrome Identification and Treatment*) (1602 AD) by Wang Ken-tang. This citation pointed out that *Bai bi* specified the symptom of white-coloured scales, while *She shi* is the name of the condition. This condition was described as 'white-coloured skin lesion all over the whole body of various sizes and shapes, with itchiness but no pain; white scales appears after scratching'. This passage was also cited by several books from the Qing dynasty such as *Yang Yi Da Quan* (*Complete Collection of Skin Diseases*) (1760 AD), which confirmed that *Bai bi* referred to white-coloured scales, while *She shi* was the name of the condition. Another Ming dynasty book, *Wai Ke Zheng Zhi Quan Shu* (*Complete Collection of the Pattern/Syndrome Identification and Treatment of External Medicine*) (1831 AD) stated that *Bi feng* was actually an alternative name of *Bai bi* — a condition with symptoms of dry and itchy skin with white-coloured lesions and scales that appear after scratching.

Syndromes of Psoriasis Vulgaris in Classical Literature

The aetiology of *Bai bi* was described in the citation as:

'Bai bi appears on the skin all over the body, shaped like Jie or Zhen, white in colour and itchy; scratching will make white-coloured scales. This is caused by external wind invading the skin, internal Blood-dryness causing lack of nourishment of the skin' (in the book *Tong Yuan Yi Shu Wai Ke*, 1881 AD).

She shi was also another term for *Bai bi*:

'She shi is an alternative name of Bai bi; it appears on the skin all over the body, shaped-like Jie or Zhen, white in colour and itchy; scratching will make white-coloured scales. This is caused by external wind invading the skin, internal Blood-dryness causing lack of nourishment of the skin' (in the book *Wai Ke Bei Yao*, 1904 AD).

Bi feng was also an alternative term of *Bai bi*:

'In Bai bi (also named Bi feng), the skin is dry and itchy, firstly appearing like Jie or Zhen. Scratching will make scales; after a long time the skin will become dry, lacking in nourishment, cracked and bleeding and will cause pain; the skin between ten fingers will become thick and difficult to scratch. The disease is caused by severe dryness in late autumn season. It is often seen in people who have Blood deficiency and are thin in body shape' (in the book *Wai Ke Zheng Zhi Quan Shu*, 1831 AD).

Therefore, the aetiology of *Bai bi, Bi feng* and *She shi* was believed to be external wind invasion in combination with Blood deficiency and dryness as the internal factor.

Common Formulae and Herbs

Among the 60 most likely psoriasis vulgaris citations, a total of seven named orally used formulae and 15 topically used formulae were found. A total of 56 different herbs were contained in the seven oral formulae while 69 different herbs were in the 15 topical formulae. Table 3.2 presents the formulae recommended by multiple citations, and Table 3.3 presents the top 10 most frequently used herb ingredients of all formulae among these 60 citations.

Table 3.2   Most Frequently Used Formulae in Classical Literature

Orally Used Formulae			Topically Used Formulae		
Formula Name	Citations	Herb Ingredients	Formula Name	Citations	Herb Ingredients
Sou feng shun qi wan	5	*Da huang, jiu, shan yao, da zao, niu xi, tu si zi, zhi ke, yu li ren, qiang huo, fang feng, du huo, che qian zi, bing lang, feng mi*	*Fu zi san*	2	*Fu zi, liu huang, cang er zi,*
Fang feng tong sheng san	3	*Fang feng, chuan xiong, dang gui, shao yao, da huang, bo he, ma huang, lian qiao, mang xiao, shi gao, huang qin, jie geng, hua shi, gan cao, jing jie, bai zhu, zhi zi*	*Jiang can san*	2	*Man jing zi, huang qi, fu ling, ren shen, tian nan xing, tian ma, jiang can, du huo, qiang huo, ge gen, gan cao, jing jie, etc.*

(Continued)

Table 3.2   (*Continued*)

Orally Used Formulae			Topically Used Formulae		
Formula Name	Citations	Herb Ingredients	Formula Name	Citations	Herb Ingredients
Ku shen wan	2	Ku shen, zao jiao	Yi mo san	2	Tian nan xing, cao wu tou, yang ti gen
La fan wan	2	Huang la, ming fan, zhu sha	Hai ai tang	2	Ai cao, ju hua, bo he, fang feng, hao ben, huo xiang, gan song, man jing zi, jing jie sui
Zhu shen san	2	Fu zi, jiao hong, zhu shen, yan			

Table 3.3   Most Frequently Used Herbs in Classical Literature

Orally Used Herbs		Topically Used Herbs	
Herb Name in *Pinyin*	No. of Citations	Herb Name in *Pinyin*	No. of Citations
Da huang	10	Wu tou	13
Chen jiu	10	Zhu you	9
Feng mi	9	Cu	8
Fang feng	8	Ban Mao	6
Yu li ren	7	Yang ti gen	6
Qiang huo	7	Shi liu huang	5
Zhi shi	7	She chuang zi	5
Da ma ren	7	Huang lian	4
Tu si zi	7	Zao jia or Zao jiao	4
Du huo	6	Bai fan	4

Common Acupuncture Points

There was no acupuncture treatment found amongst the 60 citations most likely considered to be psoriasis vulgaris. Nine citations introduced the technique of needling LI11 *Quchi*, which could be the treatment for *Feng xuan*. They were extracted from different acupuncture books written in the Ming or Qing dynasty or Minguo period. However, no detailed information of *Feng xuan* was given by these citations, so they were not included in the pool of terms most likely to be psoriasis vulgaris. Therefore the historical use of LI11 *Quchi* for psoriasis vulgaris is uncertain.

Classical Literature in Perspective

The results of the classical literature searched using 'ZHYD' suggested that not only *Bai bi*, but also *She shi* and *Bi feng* were the terms that most closely corresponded to psoriasis vulgaris. These three terms all first appeared in the Ming dynasty. Other terms, such as *Bai xuan*, *Feng xuan* and *Gan xuan*, which date back to before the Tang dynasty (before 618 AD), can refer to conditions consistent with psoriasis, but can also refer to diseases that are unlikely to have been psoriasis.

The aetiology of *Bai bi*, *She shi* and *Bi feng* was external wind invasion in combination with Blood deficiency and dryness as the internal factor. This is similar to the syndrome of psoriasis vulgaris in the contemporary literature. However, the Blood heat and Blood stasis syndrome was not found to be related to psoriasis vulgaris in the classical literature.

Formulae and herbs found in the most likely psoriasis vulgaris citations were also identified. Some of the formulae were inconsistent with current clinical practice. For example, some formulae are used in current practice but not as the key formula for psoriasis vulgaris (*Fang feng tong sheng san* and *Sou feng shun qi wan*), while other formulae do not exist in current practice (*Hai ai tang*, *Zhu shen san* and *Yi mo san*) and yet others are not used for psoriasis in current practice (e.g. *Yi sao guang* is used for tinea pedis in current practice).

The frequently used oral herbs in citations most likely to be psoriasis vulgaris include herbs for expelling wind (*fang feng*), removing dampness (*qiang huo, du huo* and *che qian zi*), eliminating heat (*da huang, huang qin* and *zhi zi*) and herbs for tonifying the Spleen and Kidney (*tu si zi, niu xi, shan zhu yu* and *shan yao*), while the Blood syndrome herbs commonly used in current practice for psoriasis were not the most commonly seen in the classical literature (e.g. *dang gui, chuan xiong* and *bai shao* were cited less frequently). This might be caused by the historical development of CM aetiology of this disease. In the Sui and Tang dynasties, it was believed that psoriasis was caused by external wind invasion; until the Ming and Qing dynasties, the internal factor of Blood syndrome started to be taken into consideration. Current clinical practice has a focus on Blood syndromes, especially Blood stasis.

The herbs used topically which were identified from the classical literature are more consistent with current practice. For instance, *huang lian, she chuang zi, shi liu huang, bo he* and *fang feng* are also commonly used in current practice for eliminating heat or stopping itch, and *cu* (vinegar) and *zhu you* (pig fat) are used as a dissolvent for making topical preparations. *Jin tuo* (saliva) was seen in the classical literature but is no longer in current use. In addition, toxic herbs such as *wu tou, ban mao, qian dan* and *shui yin* are rarely used in current clinical practice for the treatment of psoriasis, suggesting a limited understanding of the condition and herb toxicity in history.

Besides CHM, acupuncture was rarely used in history for the management of psoriasis-type conditions.

References

1. Ma K-W. (2000) Acupuncture: Its place in the history of Chinese medicine. *Acupunct Med* **18**(2): 88–99.
2. White A, Ernst E. (2004) A brief history of acupuncture. *Rheumatology* **43**(5): 662–663.
3. May BH, Lu Y, Lu C, Zhang AL, Chang S, Xue CC. (2013) Systematic assessment of the representativeness of published collections of the traditional literature on Chinese medicine. *J Altern Complement Med* **19**(5): 403–409.

4. May BH, Lu C, Xue CC. (2012) Collections of traditional Chinese medical literature as resources for systematic searches. *J Altern Complement Med* **18**(12): 1101–1107.
5. Chinese Academy of Chinese Medical Sciences. (2011) *Evidence-Based Guidelines of Clinical Practice in Chinese Medicine* [in Chinese: 中医循证临床实践指南]. Chinese Academy of Chinese Medical Sciences Publishing House, Beijing, People's Republic of China.
6. Zhang Y. (2009) 白疕的古文献研究浅识 [in Chinese]. *J Changchun Univ Tradit Chin Med* **25**(6): 974–975.
7. Lin XR. (2002) 隋代到清代中医医籍中有关银屑病的资料综述 [in Chinese]. *Chin J Dermatovenereol Integr Tradit West Med* **1**(1): 60–62.

4

Methods for Evaluating Clinical Evidence

Overview

The use of Chinese medicine for psoriasis vulgaris has been well described in the contemporary literature and classical Chinese literature. This section outlines the process used to identify and evaluate Chinese medicine interventions for psoriasis vulgaris in clinical studies. A comprehensive search was undertaken, with studies assessed against eligibility criteria, along with the methodological assessment of the quality of included studies. Results from included studies were analysed to provide an estimate of the effects of different Chinese medicine interventions.

Introduction

The use of Chinese medicine (CM) for psoriasis vulgaris has been well described in the contemporary literature and classical literature. Several systematic reviews have been conducted, which evaluated CM therapies for psoriasis vulgaris, including topical application of Chinese herbal medicine (CHM)[1,2] and oral application of CHM.[3-5] So far, no systematic review on acupuncture or other CM therapies for psoriasis vulgaris has been conducted.

This chapter describes the methods used to examine CM interventions for psoriasis vulgaris in clinical studies. Efficacy and safety will be examined in controlled clinical trials. Interventions have been categorised as follows:

- Chinese herbal medicine (CHM) (Chapter 5)

- Acupuncture and related therapies (Chapter 7)
- Combination of CM therapies (Chapter 8).

References to clinical trials were obtained and assessed by an expert group. References to all studies can be found in Appendix 1. Randomised controlled trials (RCTs), non-randomised controlled clinical trials (CCTs) and non-controlled studies were evaluated in detail. CCTs were evaluated using the same approach as the controlled trials, and have been described separately. Evidence from non-controlled studies is more difficult to evaluate, therefore the approach was taken to describe the characteristics of the study, details of the intervention and any adverse events.

Search Strategy

Evidence was searched in databases both in English and Chinese, where the search methods followed the *Cochrane Handbook of Systematic Reviews*.[6] Databases in English included PubMed, Embase, CINAHL, CENTRAL and AMED, and databases in Chinese included CBM, CNKI, CQVIP and Wanfang. Databases were accessed from inception to May 2013. No restrictions were applied. Search terms were mapped to controlled vocabulary (where applicable) in addition to being searched as keywords. To conduct a comprehensive search of the literature, the three search blocks for each intervention were combined using 'AND' (or database-specific variants), resulting in nine searches in each of the nine databases:

1. CHM reviews
2. CHM RCTs/CCTs
3. CHM non-controlled studies
4. Acupuncture and related therapies reviews
5. Acupuncture and related therapies RCTs/CCTs
6. Acupuncture and related therapies non-controlled studies
7. Other CM therapies reviews

8. Other CM therapies RCTs/CCTs
9. Other CM therapies non-controlled studies.

Studies of combination CM therapies were identified through the above searches. In addition to electronic databases, reference lists of systematic reviews and included studies were searched for additional publications. Clinical trials registers were examined to identify clinical trials which were ongoing or completed, and where required, trial investigators were contacted to obtain data. Trial registers included:

- Australian New Zealand Clinical Trial Registry (ANZCTR)
- Chinese Clinical Trial Registry (ChiCTR)
- EU Clinical Trials Register (EU-CTR)
- ClinicalTrials.gov

Inclusion Criteria

- Participants: people with a diagnosis of psoriasis vulgaris
- Interventions: CHM (orally or topically administration), acupuncture and related therapies, or other CM therapies (see Table 4.1)
- Comparators: placebo, no treatment, pharmacotherapies and phototherapies that are recommended by international guidelines of psoriasis

Table 4.1   Chinese Medicine Interventions Included in Clinical Evidence Evaluation

Category	Intervention
Chinese Herbal Medicine (CHM)	Oral CHM, Topical CHM
Acupuncture and related therapies	Acupuncture, acupressure, ear acupuncture, ear acupressure, electro-acupuncture, laser acupuncture, moxibustion
Other Chinese medicine therapies	Tuina (Chinese massage), cupping, medicated cupping, electro-cupping, stone acupuncture point stimulation, qigong therapy, taichi therapy, Chinese pulmonary rehabilitation, Ba duan jin (Qigong) therapy, phototherapy/infrared, Chinese medicine (CM) diet therapy, CM psychological intervention

Table 4.2   Outcome Measures Used in Clinical Studies

Outcome Categories	Outcome Measures	Unit; Direction for Improvement; Range
Change of psoriasis vulgaris symptom severity	1. PASI 60 (or above)	Number; N/A; N/A
	2. Lesion reduction (criteria of calculation is not specified) of 60%	Number; N/A; N/A
Health-related quality of life	DLQI	Points; ↓; 0–30

- Studies reported at least one of the pre-specified outcome measures (Table 4.2)

Exclusion Criteria

- Studies that included participants of other type of psoriasis; and
- Studies that applied pharmacotherapy which were not recommended by clinical practice guidelines as co-intervention or control intervention.

Methodological Quality Assessment

Risk of bias was assessed for RCTs using the Cochrane Collaboration's tool,[7] with the following domains: sequence generation, allocation concealment, blinding of participants, blinding of personnel, blinding of outcome assessors, incomplete outcome data and selective reporting. Each domain was evaluated to determine whether the risk of bias was low, high or unclear. Risk of bias assessment was verified by a second person, and disagreement was resolved by discussion or consultation with a third person.

Risk of bias is categorised using the following six domains:

- Sequence generation: method used to generate the allocation sequence is given in sufficient detail to allow an assessment of whether it should produce comparable groups. Low risk of bias refers to a random number table or computer random generator. High risk of bias includes studies that describe a non-random sequence generation such as odd or even date of birth or date of admission.

- Allocation concealment: method used to conceal the allocation sequence is given in enough detail to determine whether intervention allocations could have been foreseen before or during enrolment. Low risk of bias includes central ransomisation or sealed envelopes and high risk of bias includes open random sequence or date of birth etc.
- Blinding of participants and personnel: measures used to describe if the study participants and personnel are blind to the intervention received. In addition, information relating to whether the blinding was effective is also assessed. Studies that ensure blinding of participants and personnel are at low risk of bias. If the study is not blind or incompletely blind it is at high risk of bias.
- Blinding of outcome assessors: measures used to describe if the outcome assessors are blind from knowledge of which intervention a participant received. In addition, information relating to whether the blinding was effective is also assessed. Studies that ensure blinding of outcome assessors are at low risk of bias. If the study is not blind or incompletely blind it is at high risk of bias.
- Incomplete outcome data: completeness of outcome data for each main outcome, including drop outs and exclusions from the analysis with numbers missing in each group and reasons for drop out or exclusions. Studies with low risk of bias would include all outcome data or if there is missing data it is unlikely to relate to the true outcome or is balanced between groups. Studies at high risk of bias would have unexplained missing data.
- Selective reporting: the study protocol is available and the pre-specified outcomes are included in the report. Studies with a published protocol and include all pre-specified outcomes in their report would be at low risk of bias. Studies at high risk of bias would not include all pre-specified outcome or the outcome data is reported incompletely.

Statistical Analyses

Frequency of CM syndromes, CHM formulae, herbs and acupuncture points reported in included studies are presented using descriptive statistics. CM syndromes reported in two or more studies were presented. The 10 most frequently reported CHM formulae and 20 most frequently reported herbs are presented where used in at least two studies, although for CHM formulae this was not always possible. The top ten acupuncture points used in two or more studies are presented, or as available. Where data was limited, reports of single CM syndromes or acupuncture points were provided as a guide for the reader.

Definitions of statistical tests and results are described in Table 4.3. Dichotomous data are reported as a risk ratio (RR) with 95% confidence intervals (CI) and continuous data are reported as mean difference (MD) with 95% CI. For all analyses, the estimates of I^2 were reported with RR or MD and 95% CI. Formal tests for heterogeneity were conducted using the I^2 statistic. An I^2 score greater than 50% was considered to indicate substantial heterogeneity.[6] Sensitivity analyses were then undertaken to explore potential sources of heterogeneity. Where possible and appropriate, planned sub-group analyses included duration of the disease, severity of the disease, duration of treatment, CM syndromes and CM formulae and/or herbs. Available case analysis with a random effects model was used in all analyses. The random effects model was used to take into account the clinical heterogeneity likely to be encountered within and between included studies, and the variation in treatment effects between included studies.

Assessment Using GRADE

The Grading of Recommendations Assessment, Development and Evaluation (GRADE) approach was used to summarise the quality of evidence and results of the strength of evidence for each of the critical and important chronic urticaria outcomes. The GRADE approach summarises and rates the quality of evidence in systematic reviews

Table 4.3   Explanation of Statistical Terminology

Statistical Definitions	
Mean difference (MD)	In meta-analysis: A method used to combine measures on continuous scales, where the mean, standard deviation and sample size in each group are known. The weight given to the difference in means from each study (e.g. how much influence each study has on the overall results of the meta-analysis) is determined by the precision of its estimate of effect and, in the statistical software in RevMan and the Cochrane Database of Systematic Reviews, is equal to the inverse of the variance. This method assumes that all of the trials have measured the outcome on the same scale.
Risk ratio (RR)	The ratio of risks in two groups. In intervention studies, it is the ratio of the risk in the intervention group to the risk in the control group. A risk ratio of one indicates no difference between comparison groups. For undesirable outcomes, a risk ratio that is less than one indicates that the intervention was effective in reducing the risk of that outcome.
95% confidence interval (95% CI)	Confidence intervals around the estimate of effect from each study are one way of expressing precision, with a narrower confidence interval meaning more precision.
Effect size	A generic term for the estimate of effect of treatment for a study.

Note: All definitions are taken from the *Cochrane Handbook of Systematic Reviews.*

using a structured process for presenting evidence summaries. The results are presented in summary of findings tables. The results provide an important overview for chronic urticaria outcomes.

A panel of experts was established to evaluate the quality of evidence. The panel included the systematic review team, Chinese medicine practitioners, integrative medicine experts, research methodologists, and Western medicine physicians. Experts were asked to rate the clinical importance for key interventions in each intervention grouping (CHM, acupuncture therapies and other CM therapies), comparators and outcomes. Results were collated and, based on the mean rating score and subsequent discussion, a consensus on the content for the Summary of findings (SOF) tables was achieved.

The quality of evidence for each outcome was rated according to five factors outlined in the GRADE approach. The quality of evidence may be rated down based on:

- Limitations in study design (risk of bias)
- Inconsistency of results (unexplained heterogeneity)
- Indirectness of evidence (interventions, populations and outcomes important to the patients with the condition)
- Imprecision (uncertainty about the results)
- Publication bias (selective publication of studies)

These five factors are additive and a reduction in more than one factor will reduce the quality of the evidence for that outcome. The GRADE approach also includes three domains that can be rated up, including large magnitude of an effect, dose-response gradient and effect of plausible residual confounding. However, these three domains relate to observational studies including cohort, case-control, before-after, time series studies, etc. GRADE summaries in this monograph only include RCTs therefore these three domains for rating up were not assessed.

Treatment recommendations can also be assessed using the GRADE approach but due to the diverse nature of CM practice, treatment recommendations were not included with the summary of findings. Therefore the reader is able to interpret the evidence with reference to the local practice environment. It should also be noted that the GRADE approach requires judgments about the quality of evidence and some subjective assessment. However the experience of the panel members suggests the judgments are reliable and transparent representations of the quality of evidence.

The GRADE levels of evidence are grouped into four categories[8]:

1) High quality evidence: Further research is very unlikely to change our confidence in the estimate of effect.
2) Moderate quality evidence: Further research is likely to have an important impact on our confidence in the estimate of effect and may change the estimate.
3) Low quality evidence: Further research is very likely to have an important impact on our confidence in the estimate of effect and is likely to change the estimate.
4) Very low quality evidence: Any estimate of effect is very uncertain.

Outcome Measures

For the outcome measure, international guidelines have suggested Psoriasis Area Severity Index (PASI) 75 (a 75% reduction of PASI score) as the goal of psoriasis therapies and PASI 50 (a 50% reduction of PASI score) as the minimum treatment target.[9,10] In China, PASI 60 (a 60% reduction of PASI score) is considered by the 'Consensus on integrative medicine diagnosis and treatment of psoriasis vulgaris' as the cut-off level to measure effectiveness of treatment.[11] Clinical trials of psoriasis vulgaris conducted in China usually report the total effective rate (TER) as the primary outcome measure. The TER often is calculated based on PASI score reduction or other lesion reduction (criteria of calculation is not specified), with 90%, 60% and 30% of symptom reduction being the most commonly seen levels of effectiveness. However, when clinical studies reported the TER, participants who achieved the lowest level (usually 30%) of symptom reduction were considered as 'effective cases' and be pooled for TER calculation. This approach is inconsistent with the recognised treatment goal in accordance to international Chinese guidelines, and it may have exaggerated the treatment effect of a therapy. In order to reflect the treatment effect consistently with clinical guidelines, we selected a 60% or greater reduction of symptom (PASI score or lesion score) as the primary outcome. If any study reported 65%, 70% or 75% of symptom reduction, such data were pooled in the 60% level, following a conservative approach. In addition, Dermatology Life Quality Index (DLQI) was also used in our evaluation (Table 4.2).

References

1. Deng S, May BH, Zhang AL, Lu C, Xue CC. (2014) Topical herbal formulae in the management of psoriasis: Systematic review with meta- analysis of clinical studies and investigation of the pharmacological actions of the main herbs. *Phytother Res* **28**(4): 480–497.

2. Li N, Li YQ, Li HY, Guo W, Bai YP. (2012) Efficacy of externally applied Chinese herbal drugs in treating psoriasis: A systematic review. *Chin J Integr Med* **18**(3): 222–229.

3. May BH, Zhang AL, Zhou W, Lu CJ, Deng S, Xue CC. (2012) Oral herbal medicines for psoriasis: A review of clinical studies. *Chin J Integr Med* **18**(3): 172–178.

4. Zhang ZW, Wang JZ, Zhang H, Pang CK, Liu YX. (2003) [in Chinese]: 中草药治疗寻常型银屑病随机对照试验的循证评价.]. *Chin J Leprosy Skin Dis* **19**: 370–372.

5. Zhan QX, Xu LM. (2007) 雷公藤治疗银屑病的系统评价 [in Chinese]. *Chin J Dermatol Venereol Integr Tradit West Med* **6**: 192–196.

6. Higgins JPT, Green S, (eds). (2011) *Cochrane Handbook for Systematic Reviews of Interventions*. The Cochrane Collaboration, London.

7. Higgins JPT. (2004) The Cochrane Collaboration's tool for assessing risk of bias. The Cochrane Collaboration Retrieved from: http://ohg. cochrane.org/sites/ohg.cochrane.org/files/uploads/Risk%20of%20 bias%20assessment%20tool.pdf

8. Schünemann H, Brożek J, Guyatt G, Oxman A, (eds). (2013) *GRADE Handbook for Grading Quality of Evidence and Strength of Recommendations*. The GRADE Working Group. Retrieved from www. guidelinedevelopment.org/handbook

9. Menter A, Gottlieb A, Feldman SR, van Voorhees AS, Leonardi CL, Gordon KB, *et al.* (2008) Guidelines of care for the management of psoriasis and psoriatic arthritis: Section 1. Overview of psoriasis and guidelines of care for the treatment of psoriasis with biologics. *J Am Acad Dermatol* **58**(5): 826–850.

10. Nast A, Boehncke WH, Mrowietz U, Ockenfels HM, Philipp S, Reich K, et al. (2012) S3 — Guidelines on the treatment of psoriasis vulgaris (English version). *J Dtsch Dermatol Ges.* **10**(Suppl. 2): S1–S95.

11. Professional Committee of Dermatology of the Army Medical Association. (全军中医药学会皮肤病专业委员会). (2009) 寻常型银屑病中西医结合诊疗共识 (2009 年讨论稿) [in Chinese]. *Chin J Dermatol Venereol Integr Tradit West Med* **8**(5): 328.

5

Chinese Herbal Medicine for Psoriasis Vulgaris

Overview

Many studies published in Chinese and international scientific journals have investigated the efficacy and safety of Chinese herbal medicine (CHM) for psoriasis vulgaris. This chapter provides an up-to-date synopsis and analysis of the clinical trial literature and an assessment of the state of evidence. Comprehensive searches were conducted in nine databases, identifying over 6,300 citations. These were assessed against rigorous criteria resulting in exclusion of over 6,000 citations. Finally, 267 clinical studies that investigated CHM for psoriasis vulgaris were selected for inclusion in the analyses presented in this chapter. For the 118 included controlled clinical trials, a series of meta-analyses of results were performed to determine the efficacy and safety of oral or topical CHM for psoriasis vulgaris. The 149 non-controlled studies were evaluated to examine the interventions used and the safety profile of the CHMs tested. The evidence for CHM is promising, particularly when combined with pharmacotherapy or phototherapy.

Previous Systematic Reviews

Deng et al.[1] evaluated topical CHM formulations for psoriasis and found nine relevant studies. Eight different CHM formulations were reported. Meta-analysis revealed topical CHMs improved clinical efficacy by greater than 50% compared with topical placebo; topical pharmacotherapy alone, and topical pharmacotherapy. Scaling, induration, and itching were improved with topical CHM and there were minimal (<5%) adverse events reported in the studies. Results should be interpreted with some caution due to methodological shortfalls in the clinical trials included in the reviews and the diversity of CHM interventions investigated.

Li *et al.*[2] included 10 studies investigating topical CHMs. Interventions were prepared as CHM baths, CHM steaming therapy, and CHM ointments. CHM ingredients differed between the studies. All studies reported efficacy of their selected interventions. The review authors reported that preparations seemed to be more effective compared to UVB or placebo, but equivalent to topical Western medicine. Similar to the other reviews on topical CHMs, the included studies appeared to have methodological weakness and results need to be interpreted with caution.

Zhang *et al.*[3] evaluated the effectiveness of oral CHM for psoriasis. Nine randomised controlled trials (RCTs) with more than three months follow-up period were included. In total, 2,612 participants were included in these RCTs. Only two RCTs received a Jadad score of 3 or greater, while seven other studies scored between 0 and 2. Eight of the nine RCTs investigated CHM formulae while the ninth was for a single-herb extract. Two trials compared CHM with placebo — one trial was designed as CHM plus pharmacotherapy *vs.* pharmacotherapy alone, and the other six studies compared two CHM formulae. Adverse events reported in five studies were mild to moderate without any further details. Meta-analysis was not performed due to the heterogeneity. The author concluded that the methodological quality of included studies was poor and suggested further studies to use a double-blinded, placebo-controlled design. This review did not provide evidence of the efficacy of CHM.

Zhan *et al.*[4] evaluated the effectiveness of a single herb or compound of *Lei gong teng* for psoriasis. Nine RCTs and 819 participants were included. The Jadad scale was used to assess methodological quality of the studies but was not reported by the review. Among the nine included RCTs, five studies were designed as CHM plus pharmacotherapy *vs.* pharmacotherapy alone, one study compared CHM with placebo, while the other three studies compared CHM *Lei gong teng* to other CHM products. Meta-analysis was performed and concluded that the CHM *Lei gong teng* is more effective for psoriasis compare to control groups. There was no information of adverse events provided in this review.

Clinical Evidence: Characteristics

Chinese herbal medicine (CHM) can be administered orally or topically. Since psoriasis vulgaris is a skin condition, topical application of CHMs including CHM ointments or CHM baths were common. Oral CHMs were prescribed focusing more on the syndrome of disease while topical CHMs targeted more on the skin lesions themselves. Therefore, the evidence for oral CHMs and topical CHMs were evaluated separately.

A search databases both in English and Chinese identified 7,972 citations and duplicates accounted for 1,637 of these citations. A total of 1,048 full-text citations were screened and 781 did not meet the inclusion criteria (Figure 5.3). After exclusions, a total of 267 clinical studies are included in our systematic evaluation. Among them, there are 100 randomised controlled trials (RCTs), 18 non-randomised controlled trials (CCTs), and 149 non-controlled studies. Studies involving oral CHMs numbered 231, while 36 studies investigated topical CHMs (Figure 5.3).

Oral Chinese Herbal Medicine

In total, 75 RCTs (S1–S75; see Appendix 1), 15 CCTs (S76–S90), and 141 non-controlled studies (S91–S231) met the inclusion criteria (see Figure 5.3). Evidence of CHM for psoriasis vulgaris is available. One RCT was conducted in Hong Kong and published in English (S1); the remaining studies were conducted in mainland China and published in Chinese.

A total of 10,773 people participated in these studies. The age of the participants ranged from 11 to 70 years. The treatment duration ranged from four weeks/one month to 12 weeks/three months. Included studies investigated oral CHM compared to placebo, pharmacotherapy, phototherapy, and no treatment. In addition, included

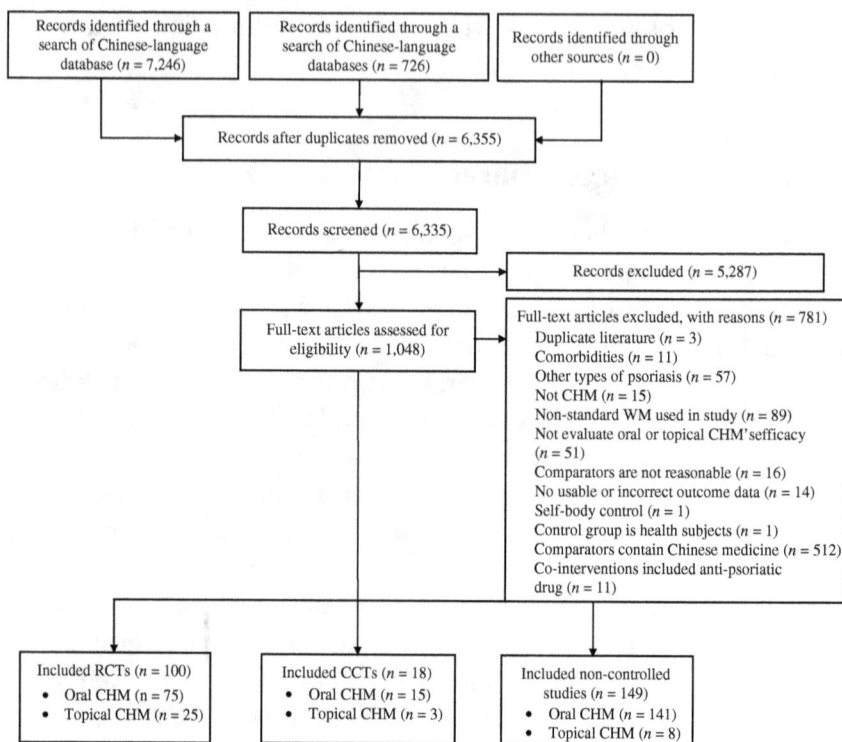

Records identified through a search of Chinese-language database ($n = 7{,}246$)	Records identified through a search of Chinese-language databases ($n = 726$)	Records identified through other sources ($n = 0$)

Records after duplicates removed ($n = 6{,}355$)

Records screened ($n = 6{,}335$)

Records excluded ($n = 5{,}287$)

Full-text articles assessed for eligibility ($n = 1{,}048$)

Full-text articles excluded, with reasons ($n = 781$)
Duplicate literature ($n = 3$)
Comorbidities ($n = 11$)
Other types of psoriasis ($n = 57$)
Not CHM ($n = 15$)
Non-standard WM used in study ($n = 89$)
Not evaluate oral or topical CHM'sefficacy ($n = 51$)
Comparators are not reasonable ($n = 16$)
No usable or incorrect outcome data ($n = 14$)
Self-body control ($n = 1$)
Control group is health subjects ($n = 1$)
Comparators contain Chinese medicine ($n = 512$)
Co-interventions included anti-psoriatic drug ($n = 11$)

Included RCTs ($n = 100$) • Oral CHM (n = 75) • Topical CHM ($n = 25$)	Included CCTs ($n = 18$) • Oral CHM ($n = 15$) • Topical CHM ($n = 3$)	Included non-controlled studies ($n = 149$) • Oral CHM ($n = 141$) • Topical CHM ($n = 8$)

Figure 5.1 Flowchart of Study Selection Process: Chinese Herbal Medicine.

studies also looked at the effects of oral CHM combined with pharmacotherapy compared to pharmacotherapy alone, or oral CHM combined with phototherapy compared to phototherapy alone. Topical pharmacotherapies included vitamin D3-analogues, corticosteroids, and tazarotene; oral pharmacotherapies included retinoids and methotrexate. Phototherapy used NB-UVB.

In total, 275 oral CHM formulae containing over 300 different herbs were tested by 231 clinical studies. Commonly seen syndromes reported in the research include Blood heat, Blood stasis, Blood dryness, and toxic heat. The most frequently tested formulas are: *Xiao yin ke li* (granule), *Run zao zhi yang jiao nang* (capsule), *Tao hong si wu tang*, and *Xi jiao di huang tang* (see Table 5.1). In addition, although some formula names [e.g., *Xiao yin yi hao fang*

Table 5.1 Summary of Oral CHM Clinical Studies

No. of Studies	No. of Participants	Most Common Syndromes (No. of Studies)	Most Common Formulae (No. of Studies)	Most Common Herbs (No. of Studies)
231	10,773	1. Blood heat ($n = 138$) 2. Blood stasis ($n = 87$) 3. Blood dryness ($n = 73$) 4. Toxic heat ($n = 38$)	1. Xiao yin ke li (granule) ($n = 6$) 2. Run zao zhi yang jiao nang (capsule) ($n = 4$) 3. Tao hong si wu tang ($n = 4$) 4. Xi jiao di huang tang ($n = 4$) 5. Dang gui yin zi ($n = 2$) 6. Liang xue jie du tang ($n = 2$) 7. Huo xue san yu tang ($n = 2$) 8. Fu fang qing dai jiao nang (capsule) ($n = 2$) 9. Pi min xiao jiao nang (capsule) ($n = 2$) 10. Ke yin yi hao fang ($n = 2$) All other formulae were not repeated in more than one study.	1. Sheng di huang ($n = 157$) 2. Dang gui ($n = 111$) 3. Chi shao ($n = 111$) 4. Dan shen ($n = 108$) 5. Tu fu ling ($n = 103$) 6. Mu dan pi ($n = 102$) 7. Bai xian pi ($n = 89$) 8. Zi cao ($n = 86$) 9. Hong hua ($n = 58$) 10. Ku shen ($n = 48$) 11. Gan cao ($n = 39$) 12. Ji xue teng ($n = 36$) 13. Da qing ye/ban lan gen/qing dai ($n = 36$) 14. Bai hua she she cao ($n = 35$) 15. Jin yin hua ($n = 32$) 16. Bai mao gen ($n = 28$) 17. Huai hua ($n = 25$) 18. He shou wu ($n = 23$) 19. Zhi zi ($n = 20$) 20. Fang feng ($n = 20$)

(*n* = 2), *Ke yin yi hao fang* (*n* = 3)] were seen in multiple studies, these formulae actually contain different ingredients and therefore were not considered as the same formulae (see Table 5.1).

Topical Chinese Herbal Medicine

Topical CHM has been researched in 25 RCTs (S232–S256), three CCTs (S257–S259), and eight non-controlled studies (S260–S267). Evidence for psoriasis is available. Most studies were conducted in mainland China, and some studies conducted in Taiwan.

Over 3,500 people participated in these studies. The age of the participants ranged from 5 to 80 years. Treatment duration for psoriasis vulgaris ranged from 20 days to 12 weeks. Research investigated topical CHM compared to placebo and pharmacotherapy. In addition, research also looked at the effects of topical CHM combined with pharmacotherapy or NB-UVB, compared to pharmacotherapy or NB-UVB alone. Pharmacotherapies included topically used vitamin D3-analogues, corticosteroids and tazarotene, and orally used retinoids and methotrexate. Phototherapy used NB-UVB.

A total of 44 different formulae and over 450 different herbs have been researched and CHMs were administered as ointment, cream, lotion, bath, fumigation or tincture/oil. Commonly reported syndromes in included studies were Blood heat, Blood dryness and Blood stasis (see Table 5.2). Three formulae were used in two studies each: *Bing huang fu le ruan gao, Di yin xi ji,* and *Yin xie gao.* There was no overlap in formulae in the remaining studies.

The database search and study selection procedure is shown in Figure 5.1.

Randomised Controlled Trials of Oral CHM

Risk of Bias Assessment

All studies were described as 'randomised'; however, only 10 studies reported an appropriate method for random sequence generation. Three studies that reported appropriate allocation concealment

Table 5.2 Summary of Topical CHM Clinical Studies

No. of Studies	No. of Participants	Most Common Syndromes (No. of Studies)	Most Common Formulae (No. of Studies)	Most Common Herbs (No. of Studies)
36	3,506	1. Blood heat (*n* = 9) 2. Blood dryness (*n* = 5) 3. Blood stasis (*n* = 5)	1. *Bing huang fu le ruan gao* (*n* = 2) 2. *Di yin xi ji* (*n* = 2) 3. *Yin xie gao* (*n* = 2) All other formulae were not repeated in more than one study.	1. *Ku shen* (*n* = 15) 2. *Bai xian pi* (*n* = 14) 3. *Hong hua* (*n* = 12) 4. *E zhu* (*n* = 12) 5. *Di fu zi* (*n* = 10) 6. *Chi shao* (*n* = 10) 7. *Dan shen* (*n* = 10) 8. *Dang gui* (*n* = 9) 9. *Huang bo* (*n* = 9) 10. *Jin yin hua* (*n* = 9) 11. *Ce bai ye* (*n* = 9) 12. *Sheng di huang* (*n* = 8) 13. *Tu fu ling* (*n* = 7) 14. *Gan cao* (*n* = 6) 15. *Yin chai hu* (*n* = 6) 16. *Hua jiao* (*n* = 6) 17. *Jing jie* (*n* = 6) 18. *Huang qin* (*n* = 6) 19. *Bing pian* (*n* = 6) 20. *Ju hua* (*n* = 5)

Table 5.3   Risk of Bias of Included RCTs: Oral CHM

Risk of Bias Domain	Low Risk *n* (%)	Unclear Risk *n* (%)	High Risk *n* (%)
Sequence generation	10 (13.3%)	52 (69.3%)	13 (17.3%)
Allocation concealment	3 (4.0%)	59 (78.7%)	13 (17.3%)
Blinding of participants	4 (5.3%)	0 (0%)	71 (94.7%)
Blinding of personnel	4 (5.3%)	0 (0%)	71 (94.7%)
Blinding of outcome assessors	0 (0%)	75 (100%)	0 (0%)
Incomplete outcome data	64 (85.3%)	1 (1.3%)	10 (13.3%)
Selective outcome reporting	0 (0%)	74 (98.7%)	1 (1.3%)

therefore were judged as 'low risk': 13 studies were 'high risk' because they allocated participants based on the order of attendance, whereas the other 59 studies were 'unclear' due to a lack of information. Blinding of participants and personnel were categorised as 'low risk' in four studies and 'high risk' in the remaining studies. All studies were 'unclear' for the blinding of outcome assessors. Incomplete outcome data was mostly at 'low risk'. In one study, selective outcome reporting was categorised as 'high risk' because pre-specified outcomes were not reported in the results, while others were 'unclear' because protocols could not be identified for any of the studies. Overall, the methodological quality was low and results should be interpreted with caution because none of the studies were free from bias (see Table 5.3 for a summary).

Effects of Oral CHM

The effects of oral CHM were assessed using PASI 60, lesion reduction of 60%, and DLQI outcome measures:

PASI 60

Many studies reported on the outcome PASI 60 or greater, and meta-analyses were possible for CHM *vs.* placebo, CHM *vs.*

pharmacotherapy as well as oral CHM used as an add-on therapy to pharmacotherapy and phototherapy (see Table 5.4).

Compared to placebo, meta-analysis showed that people who received oral CHM were 2.83 times more likely to achieve PASI 60, although statistical heterogeneity was noted ($I^2 = 60\%$). There was no statistical difference between multi-ingredient CHM and pharmacotherapy. When analyses focused on classes of pharmacotherapy, meta-analysis of nine studies of CHM *vs.* oral retinoid showed CHM was not statistically different to pharmacotherapy, while results from a single RCT showed people who received CHM were 1.4 times more likely to achieve PASI 60 than those who received topical tazarotene.

No studies were identified which compared oral CHM to phototherapy.

As an add-on therapy, oral CHM combined with pharmacotherapy was 1.28 times more likely to achieve PASI 60 than pharmacotherapy alone. Looking into particular types of pharmacotherapy, meta-analysis showed that:

- The combination of multi-ingredient oral CHM with topical vitamin D3-analogues was 1.26 times more likely to achieve PASI 60 than using topical vitamin D3-analogues alone; and
- When compared to oral retinoid alone, meta-analysis showed that combining multi-ingredient oral CHM with oral retinoid was 1.27 times more likely to achieve PASI 60 than using oral retinoid alone.

It is worth noting that two formulae have been used in multiple studies; these two formulae were proven effective as an add-on therapy:

- In two studies (S44 and S45) which used *Run zao zhi yang jiao nang* (capsule), the overall effect of the oral CHM combined with topical vitamin D3-analogues was 1.29 times more likely to achieve PASI 60 than using calcipotriol alone; and
- Two studies (S38 and S41) which used *Pi min xiao jiao nang* (capsule) showed that the combination of *Pi min xiao jiao nang* and topical vitamin D3-analogues was 1.28 times more likely to achieve PASI 60 than using calcipotriol alone.

Table 5.4 Summary of Meta-Analysis of Oral CHM for Psoriasis Vulgaris RCTs (PASI 60)

Intervention	Comparator	No. of Studies	Included Studies	Effect Size (RR [95% CI])	I^2 (%)
Oral CHM	Placebo	4	S1, S18, S20, S22	2.83 [1.23, 6.51]*	60
	Pharmacotherapy	10	S2, S5, S8–S11, S16, S19, S21, S23	1.04 [0.96, 1.13]	41
	Oral retinoid	9	S5, S8–S11, S16, S19, S21, S23	1.00 [0.95, 1.04]	0
	Add-on therapy to pharmacotherapy	21	S25, S28–S30, S32, S33, S36–S46, S49–S51, S53, S55	1.28 [1.21, 1.36]*	11
	Add-on therapy to topical vitamin D3-analogues	5	S33, S38, S41, S44, S45	1.26 [1.13, 1.39]*	0
	Add-on therapy to oral retinoid	11	S25, S29, S30, S32, S36, S37, S40, S42, S43, S49, S53	1.27 [1.14, 1.34]*	41
	Add-on therapy to phototherapy	14	S56–S58, S60–S65, S67, S68, S70–S73, S75)	1.33 [1.24, 1.44]*	5
Run zao zhi yang jiao nang	Add-on therapy to topical vitamin D3-analogues	2	S44, S45	1.29 [1.07, 1.55]*	0
Pi min xiao jiao nang	Add-on therapy to topical vitamin D3-analogues	2	S38, S41	1.28 [1.11, 1.47]*	0

*Statistically significant.

Furthermore, meta-analysis showed the combination of multi-ingredient oral CHM and phototherapy using NB-UVB was 1.33 times more likely to achieve PASI 60 than using NB-UVB alone.

Lesion Reduction of 60%

Many studies reported a reduction in lesion severity using investigator-designed criteria. No studies compared oral CHM with placebo or phototherapy. One meta-analysis showed that there was no statistical difference between multi-ingredient CHM and oral retinoid in reducing lesions, with considerable heterogeneity detected (see Table 5.5).

Nine studies (S4, S24, S26, S31, S34, S35, S47, S52 and S54) used multi-ingredient CHM as an add-on therapy to pharmacotherapy drugs. Meta-analysis showed that adding CHM to pharmacotherapy drugs was 1.31 times more likely to achieve lesion reduction of 60% than using pharmacotherapy drugs alone.

When drug class was considered, the effects of CHM varied. Meta-analysis showed that combining multi-ingredient oral CHM with oral retinoid was 1.34 times more likely to achieve lesion reduction of 60% compared to oral retinoid alone. Results from a single study showed that adding multi-ingredient oral CHM to methotrexate was 1.24 times more likely to achieve lesion reduction of 60% than methotrexate alone (RR: 1.24 [1.06, 1.44]) (S54). No benefit was found using oral CHM as an add-on therapy to other type of pharmacotherapy drugs for this outcome.

Furthermore, when adding multi-ingredient oral CHM to phototherapy using NB-UVB, meta-analysis showed that there was no significant difference between the combination and phototherapy alone, although considerable heterogeneity was detected.

Health-related Quality of Life: DLQI

Meta-analysis suggested that there was no statistical difference between multi-ingredient CHM and oral retinoid for in terms of Dermatology Life Quality Index (DLQI) score (see Table 5.6). Results

Table 5.5 Summary of Meta-Analysis of Oral CHM for Psoriasis Vulgaris RCTs (Lesion Reduction of 60%)

Intervention	Comparator	No. of Studies	Included Studies	Effect Size (RR [95% CI])	I^2 (%)
Oral CHM	Oral retinoid	5	S3, S4, S6, S7, S15	1.35 [0.94, 1.95]	68
	Add-on therapy to pharmacotherapy	9	S4, S24, S26, S31, S34, S35, S47, S52, S54	1.31 [1.20, 1.43]*	7
	Add-on therapy to oral retinoid	6	S4, S24, S26, S34, S35, S52	1.34 [1.21, 1.49]*	0
	Add-on therapy to phototherapy	2	S59, S66	1.16 [0.89, 1.51]	77

*Statistically significant.

Table 5.6 Summary of Meta-Analysis of Oral CHM for Psoriasis Vulgaris RCTs (DLQI)

Intervention	Comparator	No. of Studies	Included Studies	Effect Size (RR [95% CI])	I^2 (%)
Oral CHM	Oral retinoid	2	S12, S21	−0.60 [−1.44, 0.24]	0

from a single study showed that multi-ingredient CHM was more effective than placebo for improving patients DLQI score by 4.08 points on a 30-point scale.

Assessment Using GRADE

Three GRADE Summary of Findings (SOF) tables represent the main comparisions for oral CHM for psoriasis vulgaris, where one compares oral CHM with placebo (Table 5.7) and another compares the combination of oral CHM and oral retinoid to oral retinoid alone (Table 5.8), and the last one compares the combination of oral CHM and topical vitamin D3-analogues to topical vitamin D3-analogues alone (Table 5.9).

Evidence for oral CHM *vs.* placebo was of very low to moderate quality (Table 5.7). The result was statistically significant for PASI 60 and above, and DLQI.

Evidence for oral CHM *vs.* oral retinoid was of low quality (Table 5.8). The result was not significant for either PASI 60 and above or DLQI.

Evidence for oral CHM plus topical vitamin D3-analogues *vs.* topical vitamin D3-analogues was of moderate quality (Table 5.9). The result was significant for PASI 60 and above. DLQI was not reported by the included studies.

Frequently Reported Herbs in Meta-Analyses Showing Favourable Effect

In order to provide a list of possibly effective oral CHM herbs for the treatment of psoriasis vulgaris, all RCTs included in the meta-analyses showing favourable effect were pooled. The most frequently used herbs in these RCTs are summarised (see Table 5.10). These herbs may have contributed to the results of the effect of meta-analyses.

Table 5.7   Oral CHM vs. Placebo for Psoriasis Vulgaris SOF Table

Oral CHM Compared to Placebo for Psoriasis Vulgaris

Outcomes	No. of Participants (Studies)	Quality of Evidence (GRADE)	Relative Effect (95% CI)	Anticipated Absolute Effects	
				Risk with Placebo	Risk Difference with Chinese Herbal Medicine
PASI 60 and above Follow up: median 6 weeks (end of treatment)	234 (4 RCTs)	⊕◯◯◯ VERY LOW [1][2][3]	RR 2.83 (1.23 to 6.51)	167 per 1,000	472 per 1,000 (205 to 1,000)
DLQI Follow up: median 8 weeks (end of treatment)	62 (1 RCT)	⊕⊕⊕◯ MODERATE [4]	—	The mean DLQI in the control group was 0	The mean DLQI in the intervention group was **4.08 points lower** (7.45 points lower to 0.71 points lower)
Adverse events (AEs)	234 (4 RCTs)		Fifteen AEs were reported in intervention groups and 1 AE was reported in control groups. AEs included 15 cases of gastrointestinal symptoms and one case of menstrual disorder. All AEs were mild.		

*The risk in the intervention group (and its 95% CI) is based on the assumed risk in the comparison group and the relative effect of the intervention (and its 95% CI). CI: confidence interval; RR: risk ratio.

GRADE Working Group Grades of Evidence.

High quality: We are very confident that the true effect lies close to that of the estimate of the effect.

Moderate quality: We are moderately confident in the effect estimate: The true effect is likely to be close to the estimate of the effect, but there is a possibility that it is substantially different.

Low quality: Our confidence in the effect estimate is limited: The true effect may be substantially different from the estimate of the effect.

Very low quality: We have very little confidence in the effect estimate: The true effect is likely to be substantially different from the estimate of effect.

1. Lack of blinding of participants and personnel.
2. Considerable statistical heterogeneity.
3. The OIS criterion is not met.
4. Small sample size limits certainty of results.

Table 5.8 Oral CHM *vs.* Oral Retinoid for Psoriasis Vulgaris SOF Table

Oral CHM *vs.* Oral Retinoid for Psoriasis Vulgaris

Outcomes	No. of Participants (Studies)	Quality of Evidence (GRADE)	Relative Effect (95% CI)	Risk with Oral Retinoid	Anticipated Absolute Effects
					Risk Difference with Oral CHM Plus Oral Retinoid
PASI 60 and above Follow up: median 12 weeks (end of treatment)	1,136 (9 RCTs)	⊕⊕◯◯ LOW [1][2]	RR 1.00 (0.95 to 1.04)	723 per 1000	723 per 1,000 (687 to 752)
DLQI Follow up: range 8–12 weeks (end of treatment)	119 (2 RCTs)	⊕⊕◯◯ LOW [1][3]	—	The mean DLQI in the control group was 2.8	The mean DLQI in the intervention group was **0.6 points lower** (1.44 points lower to 0.24 points higher)
Adverse events (AEs)	1,136 (9 RCTs)		Thirty-six AEs were reported in intervention groups and 412 AEs were reported in control groups. AEs reported by the intervention groups were mainly mild gastrointestinal symptoms; AEs reported by the control groups were mainly the commonly seen AEs caused by oral retinoids, including dry mouth, dry skin, itching, hand desquamation, cheilitis, increased liver enzyme, increased blood lipids, etc.		

*The risk in the intervention group (and its 95% CI) is based on the assumed risk in the comparison group and the relative effect of the intervention (and its 95% CI).

CI: confidence interval; RR: risk ratio.

GRADE Working Group Grades of Evidence.

High quality: We are very confident that the true effect lies close to that of the estimate of the effect.

Moderate quality: We are moderately confident in the effect estimate: The true effect is likely to be close to the estimate of the effect, but there is a possibility that it is substantially different.

Low quality: Our confidence in the effect estimate is limited: The true effect may be substantially different from the estimate of the effect.

Very low quality: We have very little confidence in the effect estimate: The true effect is likely to be substantially different from the estimate of effect.

1. Lack of blinding of participants and personnel.
2. Publication bias suspected.
3. Small sample size limits certainty of results.

Table 5.9 Oral CHM plus Topical Vitamin D3-Analogues vs. Topical Vitamin D3-Analogues for Psoriasis Vulgaris SOF Table

Oral CHM plus Topical Vitamin D3-Analogues vs. Topical Vitamin D3-Analogues

Outcomes	No. of Participants (Studies)	Quality of Evidence (GRADE)	Relative Effect (95% CI)	Anticipated Absolute Effects	
				Risk with Calcipotriol	Risk Difference with Oral CHM Plus Calcipotriol
PASI 60 and above Follow up: median 12 weeks (end of treatment)	442 (5 RCTs)	⊕⊕⊕◯ MODERATE[1]	RR 1.26 (1.13 to 1.39)	689 per 1,000	868 per 1,000 (778 to 957)
DLQI not reported	—	—	—	—	—
Adverse events (AEs)	442 (5 RCTs)	Mild skin irritation was reported by both groups, and studies concluded that those AEs were caused by the topical vitamin D3-analogues.			

*The risk in the intervention group (and its 95% CI) is based on the assumed risk in the comparison group and the relative effect of the intervention (and its 95% CI).

CI: confidence interval; RR: risk ratio.

GRADE Working Group Grades of Evidence.

High quality: We are very confident that the true effect lies close to that of the estimate of the effect.

Moderate quality: We are moderately confident in the effect estimate: The true effect is likely to be close to the estimate of the effect, but there is a possibility that it is substantially different.

Low quality: Our confidence in the effect estimate is limited: The true effect may be substantially different from the estimate of the effect.

Very low quality: We have very little confidence in the effect estimate: The true effect is likely to be substantially different from the estimate of effect.

1. Lack of blinding of participants and personnel.

Table 5.10 Frequently Used Herbs in Meta-Analyses of Oral CHM for Psoriasis Vulgaris RCTs Showing Favourable Effect

Outcome	No. of Meta-Analyses	No. of Studies	Herbs (No. of Studies Using the Herb)
PASI 60	3	41	1. *Sheng di huang* (29 studies) 2. *Tu fu ling* (20 studies) 3. *Dang gui* (17 studies) 4. *Chi shao* (17 studies) 5. *Mu dan pi* (17 studies) 6. *Ku shen* (16 studies) 7. *Bai xian pi* (16 studies) 8. *Dan shen* (16 studies) 9. *Zi cao* (15 studies) 10. *Jin yin hua* (11 studies)
Lesion reduction of 60%	1	9	1. *Sheng di huang* (8 studies) 2. *Dan shen* (5 studies) 3. *Dang gui* (5 studies) 4. *Tu fu ling* (4 studies) 5. *Chi shao* (4 studies) 6. *Mu dan pi* (4 studies) 7. *Bai xian pi* (4 studies) 8. *Ji xue teng* (3 studies) 9. *Jin yin hua* (2 studies) 10. *Gan cao* (2 studies)

Safety of Oral CHM in Randomised Controlled Trials

Three studies concluded that CHM did not cause any adverse events (AEs). Other studies reported mild AEs caused by CHM including gastrointestinal symptoms ($n = 62$), hyperlipemia ($n = 23$), dry mouth/skin ($n = 18$), and dizziness ($n = 3$). All these AEs were relieved by reducing dosage. No serious AEs were found in any of the studies.

Other AEs caused by pharmacotherapy drugs or phototherapy were also reported. Nine studies concluded that CHM caused fewer AEs than pharmacotherapy drugs in the treatment of psoriasis vulgaris. Nineteen RCTs reported that AEs in the intervention groups were fewer than those in the control groups and concluded that adding CHM could reduce the number and severity of AEs caused by pharmacotherapy drugs.

Overall, oral CHM is well tolerated and is safe for psoriasis vulgaris patients. In addition, using oral CHM as an add-on therapy may be beneficial for relieving some AEs caused by pharmacotherapy drugs or phototherapy in clinical practice.

Controlled Clinical Trials (Non-Randomised) of Oral CHM

Oral CHM has been researched in 15 CCTs (S76–S90) involving 1,919 participants with psoriasis vulgaris. These studies were all designed differently and the herbal formulae/ingredients tested by these studies were diverse, with only one CHM product (*Xiao yin ke li* granule) being evaluated in two studies.

Meta-analysis for the outcome PASI 60 showed that oral CHM was more effective than oral retinoids. Consistent with results seen in RCTs, adding oral CHM significantly increased the effectiveness of oral retinoid, and that of phototherapy using NB-UVB (see Table 5.11). Mild gastrointestinal AEs were reported caused by CHM but no medical intervention/therapy was required. It was also

Table 5.11   Summary of Meta-Analysis of Oral CHM for Psoriasis Vulgaris CCTs (PASI 60)

Intervention	Comparator	No. of Studies	Included Studies	Effect Size (RR [95% CI])	I^2 (%)
Oral CHM	Oral retinoid	2	S76, S77	RR 1.25 [1.06, 1.46]*	0
	Add-on therapy to pharmacotherapy	5	S77, S82–S85	RR: 1.32 [1.09, 1.60]*	56
	Add-on therapy to phototherapy	3	S88–S90	RR: 3.40 [1.77, 6.54]*	0

*Statistically significant.

reported that adding oral CHM could reduce the AEs caused by pharmacology drugs.

Non-Controlled Studies of Oral CHM

Furthermore, a total of 141 non-controlled clinical studies (S91–S231) were found in the search. The total number of participants was 15,280, with the largest sample size numbering 575. The type of oral CHM tested by these studies differed greatly. Major syndromes involved in the included studies are: Blood heat, Blood stasis, Blood dryness, toxic heat, wind-heat, damp-heat, Blood deficiency, or combinations of the above. The most frequently used herbs in all formulae are *sheng di huang, dang gui, chi shao, tu fu ling,* and *dan shen.* Mild AEs were reported in 37 studies, including gastrointestinal symptoms ($n = 357$), insomnia ($n = 78$), and dizziness ($n = 26$). No serious AEs caused by oral CHM were reported. The adverse events seen in non-controlled studies are consistent with those described in RCTs and CCTs.

Randomised Controlled Trials of Topical CHM

Risk of Bias Assessment

All 25 studies were described as 'randomised'; however, only four studies reported an appropriate method for random sequence generation. Three studies reported inappropriate allocation concealment therefore were categorised as 'high risk', while the remaining studies were 'unclear' due to lack of information. Blinding of participants was deemed 'low risk' of bias in one study, 'unclear' for two studies, and 'high risk' of bias in other studies. All studies were 'unclear' for the blinding of outcome assessors. Incomplete outcome data was categorised as 'low risk' of bias for all studies. Selective outcome reporting was deemed 'unclear' because protocols could not be identified for any of the studies. Overall, the methodological quality was low and results should be interpreted with caution because none of the studies were free from bias (see Table 5.12 for a summary).

Table 5.12   Risk of Bias of Included RCTs: Topical CHM

Risk of Bias Domain	Low Risk *n* (%)	Unclear Risk *n* (%)	High Risk *n* (%)
Sequence generation	4 (16%)	18 (72%)	3 (12%)
Allocation concealment	0 (0%)	22 (88%)	3 (12%)
Blinding of participants	1 (4%)	2 (8%)	22 (88%)
Blinding of personnel	1 (4%)	2 (8%)	22 (88%)
Blinding of outcome assessors	0 (0%)	25 (100%)	0 (0%)
Incomplete outcome data	25 (100%)	0 (0%)	0 (0%)
Selective outcome reporting	0 (0%)	25 (100%)	0 (0%)

Effects of Topical CHM

PASI 60

None of the included studies compared topical CHM with placebo. Compared with pharmacotherapy (tretinoin cream) alone, no benefit of topical CHM was found in a single RCT (S232) (RR: 1.07 [0.38, 3.06]).

As an add-on therapy, meta-analysis showed topical CHM did not improve PASI 60 compared with using pharmacotherapy alone (see Table 5.13). Results from a single study (S233) found the combination therapy (CHM ointment plus tazarotene gel) was 1.26 times more likely to achieve PASI 60 than using tazarotene gel alone (RR: 1.26 [1.03, 1.53]). No benefit of adding topical CHM to clobetasol cream was found in one study (S234), or when CHM was added to methotrexate and salicylic acid in another study (S235).

As an add-on therapy to NB-UVB, meta-analysis showed that combining topical CHM with phototherapy was 1.29 times more likely to achieve PASI 60 than using phototherapy alone (S236–S251) (see Table 5.13).

Analysis of different forms of topical CHM showed that people who received the combination of CHM steaming therapy and phototherapy (S241, S242, S249–S251) or CHM bath and phototherapy (S236, S238, S240, S243–S246) were 1.30 and 1.25 times more

Table 5.13   Summary of Meta-Analysis of Topical CHM for Psoriasis Vulgaris RCTs (PASI 60)

Intervention	Comparator	No. of Studies	Included Studies	Effect Size (RR [95% CI])	I^2 (%)
Topical CHM	Add-on therapy to pharmacotherapy	3	S233–S235	1.15 [0.98, 1.35]	70
	Add-on therapy to phototherapy	16	S236–S251	1.29 [1.23, 1.35]*	0
CHM steaming therapy	Add-on therapy to phototherapy	5	S241, S242, S249–S251	1.30 [1.19, 1.43]*	0
CHM bath	Add-on therapy to phototherapy	7	S236, S238, S240, S243–S246	1.25 [1.17, 1.33]*	0

*Statistically significant.

likely to achieve PASI 60 than those who received phototherapy alone, respectively.

Lesion Reduction of 60%

Compared with placebo, a single study (S252) found that people who received CHM ointment were 4.50 times more likely to achieve lesion reduction of 60% than those who received placebo (RR: 4.50 [2.34, 8.65]).

When topical CHM was compared with pharmacotherapy, meta-analysis showed that topical CHM was 2.61 times more likely to achieve lesion reduction of 60% than using pharmacotherapy alone (S253 and S254) (see Table 5.14).

As an add-on therapy, results from single study (S255) showed that people who received the combination of topical CHM ointment and compound flumetasone ointment were 1.55 times more likely to achieve lesion reduction of 60% than those who received the pharmacotherapy alone. The people who received the combination of CHM bath with NB-UVB and acitretin was 1.32 times more likely to achieve lesion reduction of 60% than those who received NB-UVB and acitretin alone (S256).

Assessment Using GRADE

One GRADE SOF table represents the main comparisons for topical CHM for psoriasis vulgaris. This compared topical CHM plus NB-UVB to NB-UVB (Table 5.15). The evidence of this comparison was of low quality. The result showed that the combination of CHM and NB-UVB was significantly more effective than NB-UVB.

Table 5.14 Summary of Meta-Analysis of Topical CHM for Psoriasis Vulgaris RCTs (Lesion Reduction of 60%)

Intervention	Comparator	No. of Studies	Included Studies	Effect Size (RR [95% CI])	I^2 (%)
Topical CHM	Pharmacotherapy	2	S253, S254	2.61 [1.75, 3.90]*	0

*Statistically significant.

Table 5.15 Topical CHM plus NB-UVB vs. NB-UVB

Topical CHM plus NB-UVB vs. NB-UVB

Outcomes	No. of Participants (Studies)	Quality of Evidence (GRADE)	Relative Effect (95% CI)	Anticipated Absolute Effects	
				Risk with NB-UVB	Risk difference with topical CHM plus NB-UVB
PASI 60 and above Follow up: median 7 weeks (end of treatment)	1,867 (16 RCTs)	⊕⊕◯◯ LOW[1][2]	**RR 1.29** (1.23 to 1.35)	686 per 1,000	886 per 1,000 (845 to 927)
DLQI Not reported	—	—	—	—	—
Adverse events (AEs)	1,867 (16 RCTs)		Skin dryness, burning sensation or pain was reported by both groups, with fewer events in the intervention groups than in the control groups. Studies concluded that those AEs were caused by the NB-UVB and adding topical CHM could reduce such AEs.		

*The risk in the intervention group (and its 95% CI) is based on the assumed risk in the comparison group and the relative effect of the intervention (and its 95% CI).

CI: confidence interval; RR: risk ratio.

GRADE Working Group Grades of Evidence.

High quality: We are very confident that the true effect lies close to that of the estimate of the effect.

Moderate quality: We are moderately confident in the effect estimate: The true effect is likely to be close to the estimate of the effect, but there is a possibility that it is substantially different.

Low quality: Our confidence in the effect estimate is limited: The true effect may be substantially different from the estimate of the effect.

Very low quality: We have very little confidence in the effect estimate: The true effect is likely to be substantially different from the estimate of effect.

1. Lacking of blinding of participants and personnel.
2. Publication bias strongly suspected.

Frequently Reported Herbs in Meta-Analyses Showing Favourable Effect

In order to provide a list of possibly effective topical CHM herbs for the treatment of psoriasis vulgaris, all RCTs included in the meta-analyses showing favourable effect were pooled. The most frequently used herbs in these RCTs are summarised (see Table 5.16). These herbs may have contributed to the effect of meta-analyses results.

Safety of Topical CHM in Randomised Controlled Trials

Adverse events were reported in three studies, which compared topical CHM with pharmacotherapy, and all studies using topical CHM as an add-on therapy. In studies which compared topical CHM to pharmacotherapy drugs, AEs caused by topical CHM involved mild skin irritation ($n = 16$); no serious AEs were reported. When combining topical CHM with pharmacotherapy drugs, all RCTs reported that AEs were caused by the pharmacotherapy drugs, with one study suggesting that adding topical CHM could

Table 5.16 Frequently Used Herbs in Meta-Analyses of Topical CHM for Psoriasis Vulgaris RCTs Showing Favourable Effect for Psoriasis

Outcome	No. of Meta-Analyses	No. of Studies	Herbs (No. of Studies Using the Herb)
PASI 60	2	12	1. *Ku shen* (7 studies) 2. *Dang gui* (5 studies) 3. *E zhu* (4 studies) 4. *Jin yin hua* (4 studies) 5. *Ce bai ye* (4 studies) 6. *Bai xian pi* (3 studies) 7. *Di fu zi* (3 studies) 8. *Sheng di huang* (2 studies) 9. *Huang bo* (2 studies)

reduce the number and severity of AEs. In these studies, the AEs reported often matched the known profile of the pharmacotherapy. When combining topical CHM with NB-UVB, 16 of the 17 RCTs reported AEs were caused by NB-UVB, and five of these studies suggested that adding topical CHM could reduce the common AEs seen with NB-UVB. Overall, the topical CHMs were safe for the treatment of psoriasis vulgaris.

Controlled Clinical Trials (Non-Randomised) of Topical CHM

Topical CHM has been researched in three studies of CCTs. There was diversity in study design and the types of herbal formulae varied. All three studies were conducted in hospitals in China and included 394 people with psoriasis vulgaris. One meta-analysis of two studies (S257 and S258) found that combined CHM bath and oral acitretin was more effective than using acitretin alone in terms of PASI 60 (see Table 5.17). One study (S259) that combined CHM bath and NB-UVB found the combination therapy was more effective than the NB-UVB alone in terms of PASI 60 (RR 1.47 [1.03, 2.09]). AEs were reported in two studies, which matched the known profile of both pharmacotherapy and NB-UVB. Both authors stated that topical CHM could reduce the AEs associated with the comparators. None of the included studies reported any AEs caused by topical CHM.

Table 5.17   Summary of Meta-Analysis of Topical CHM for Psoriasis Vulgaris CCTs (PASI 60)

Intervention	Comparator	No. of Studies	Included Studies	Effect Size (RR [95% CI])	I^2 (%)
Topical CHM bath	Add-on therapy to pharmacotherapy (acitretin)	2	S257, S258	1.34 [1.11, 1.63]*	0

*Statistically significant.

Non-Controlled Studies of Topical CHM

Eight non-controlled studies using topical CHM as the intervention were included (S260–S267). The total number of participants was 359 with the largest sample size of 106. The treatment duration was from 2 weeks to 90 days. CHM formulae used by these eight non-controlled studies were all different. The preparation forms of CHM formulae included CHM steaming therapy (two studies), CHM ointment (four studies), CHM powder (one study), and CHM oil (one study). The ingredients of the formulae all differed. AEs were not reported in any of the studies.

Summary of Chinese Herbal Medicine Clinical Evidence

Both orally or topically administered CHM showed benefits in terms of clinically relevant outcomes for psoriasis vulgaris. There has since been more research investigating the effectiveness of oral CHM compared to that of topical CHM. The Chinese medicine syndrome approach was often taken into consideration in oral CHM research; however this is not common in topical CHM research.

Outcome measures used by clinical research varied. Briefly, oral CHM is not inferior to common pharmacotherapy or phototherapy (NB-UVB), and both oral CHM and topical CHM are effective add-on therapies to common pharmacotherapy or phototherapy (NB-UVB). CHM, when combined with or phototherapy, improves psoriasis vulgaris outcomes in terms of PASI 60 or lesion reduction of 60%. There is insufficient evidence supporting CHM in improving the quality of life of patients suffering from psoriasis vulgaris. CHM is generally safe and as an add-on therapy, it may reduce common AEs caused by pharmacotherapy or phototherapy.

Furthermore, although some studies included a follow-up phase and investigated the "relapse rate", the long-term effects of both oral and topical CHM were not confirmed due to the lack of validated outcome measures being used by these studies.

Nevertheless, such results should be interpreted with caution. Most evidence was assessed to be of 'low' or 'very low' quality.

In particular, since most of the controlled studies compared CHM to conventional therapy, or compared the combination of CHM with conventional therapy to conventional therapy alone, blinding of participants or research personnel was not addressed in the trial design. Lack of blinding might have inflated the favourable effects towards CHM, considering all these studies were conducted among Chinese population.

There was a diverse range of CHM formulae and herbs evaluated. Although formula names varied greatly, common herbs were found among these formulae. The most frequently used individual herbs, firstly, are those with the Chinese medicine functions of nourishing, invigorating or cooling Blood, such as: *sheng di huang, dang gui, chi shao, dan shen,* and *mu dan pi.* These results are consistent with the syndrome types seen in contemporary literature (see Chapter 2), which suggests that psoriasis vulgaris should be treated from the perspective of Blood syndromes. Secondly, the treatment principle of "clearing heat" may also play an important role in the clinical management of psoriasis vulgaris, because "cooling" herbs such as *sheng di huang, mu dan pi, zi cao, ku shen,* and *jin yin hua* are among the most frequently used ones in clinical research. Thirdly, some herbs usually used for reducing itch, such as *di fu zi, bai xian pi,* and *tu fu ling,* are also common.

In addition, some frequently used herbs were summarised from the studies included in positive meta-analyses. These are: *sheng di huang, tu fu ling, dang gui, chi shao, mu dan pi, ku shen, bai xian pi, dan shen, zi cao,* and *jin yin hua* for oral use; and *ku shen, dang gui, e zhu, jin yin hua, ce bai ye, bai xian pi, di fu zi, sheng di huang,* and *huang bo* for topical use. Practitioners may consider these herbs when preparing CHM prescriptions for patients with psoriasis vulgaris.

References

1. Deng S, May BH, Zhang AL, Lu C, Xue CC. (2014) Topical herbal formulae in the management of psoriasis: Systematic review with meta-analysis of clinical studies and investigation of the pharmacological actions of the main herbs. *Phytother Res* **28**(4): 480–497.

2. Li N, Guo W, Li HY, Zhao WB, Bai YP. (2012) *Conference Proceedings of the National Integrative Dermatology Conference.* China Society of Integrated Traditional Chinese and Western Medicine, Beijing, People's Republic of China. Retrieved from http://cpfd.cnki.com.cn/Area/CPFDCONFArticleList-ZGZP201204002-1.htm

3. Zhang JW, Wang JZ, Zhang H, Pang CK, Liu YX. (2003) 中草药治疗寻常型银屑病随机对照试验的循证评 [in Chinese]. *Chin J Leprosy Skin Dis* **19**: 370–372.

4. Zhan QX, Xu LM. (2007) 雷公藤治疗银屑病的系统评价 [in Chinese]. *Chin J Dermatol Venereol Integr Tradit West Med* **6**: 192–196.

6

Pharmacological Actions of the Common Herbs

It is likely that the effects on psoriasis vulgaris reported in the clinical trials were mediated by phytochemical constituents of the herbs. Of the orally and topically administered herbs used, the following 11 are those most frequently applied in the clinical trials: *sheng di huang, dang gui, chi shao, dan shen, tu fu ling, mu dan pi, bai xian pi, zi cao, gan cao, ku shen* and *di fu zi*.

The findings of *in vitro* and *in vivo* experimental studies of these herbs and/or their phytochemical constituents are summarised below in relation to their effects on inflammation and proliferation and wound healing, which may account for the effects of herbs reported in clinical studies of psoriasis vulgaris.

Experimental Studies of *sheng di huang*

More than 30 compounds have been isolated from the *Rehmannia glutinosa* root with the iridoid glycoside catalpol having the highest content.[1] *Di huang* has been reported to exert anti-inflammatory and antiproliferative effects.[2-4]

A water extract of *sheng di huang* decreased the production of intracellular reactive oxygen species (ROS) induced by advanced glycation end products (AGEs) without a change in the viability of THP-1 cells. The extract dose-dependently degraded cytosolic IκB-α and the nuclear localisation of NF-κB p65. It suppressed the expression of TNF-α, COX-2 monocyte chemotactic protein-1 and I-10 (interferon gamma-induced protein 10). The extract also down-regulated the expression of RAGEs (receptor for advanced glycation end products) and the mRNA expression of RAGE.[5] In murine macrophage RAW264.7 cells, a fraction of an extract of *Rehmannia glutinosa*, which contained rehmapicrogenin and cinnamic acid, suppressed NO production and inhibit the gene and protein expression of iNOS. In lipopolysaccharide (LPS)-stimulated macrophages, this fraction down-regulated PGE2, IL-6 and COX-2.[6]

Catalpol has been reported to promoted growth of the granular layer of mouse tail scale epidermis and in a guinea pig ear model of a psoriasis-like lesion induced by propranolol, catalpol inhibited epidermal proliferation.[7]

These studies suggest that extracts of *di huang* show anti-inflammatory effects and its constituent catalpol appears to exert antiproliferative effects.

Experimental Studies of *dang gui*

In vitro and *in vivo* studies have reported that *dang gui* extract and its constituent compound ferulic acid have shown anti-inflammatory activity.[2]

Extracts of *dang gui* and *ku shen* were both found to reduce protein expression of COX-2 in a rat model of endotoxin-induced uveitis (EIU), but there was greater reduction from the combined extract which also reduced NF-κB, ICAM-1 and iNOS.[8]

In psoriasis-like lesions induced in guinea pig ears by topical propranolol, injection of an angelica polysaccharide extracted from *dang gui*, increased the apoptotic index and decreased the expression level of proliferating cell nuclear antigen (PCNA) compared to control.[9,10]

Experimental Studies of *chi shao*

Chi shao derived from the root of *Paeonia lactiflora* or *Paeonia veitchii* has been reported to show anti-inflammatory activity.[2]

The compound 1,2,3,4,6-penta-O-galloyl-beta-D-glucose (PGG), originating from methanol extracts of the *Paeonia lactiflora* root, significantly inhibited LPS-induced NO production and iNOS activity in mouse macrophages (RAW 264.7 cells) and dose-dependently inhibited COX-2 but not COX-1 activity.[11] In a human dermal micro-vascular endothelial cell line, peoniflorin from the *Paeonia lactiflora* root was found to attenuate TNF-α-induced chemokine mRNA expression, reduce the up-regulation by TNF-α of the phosphorylation of IKKB-α and extracellular signal-regulated kinase (ERK)1/2, and inhibit translocation of NF-κB to the nucleus. The study concluded that peoniflorin possessed an anti-inflammatory ability against TNF-α-induced chemokine production.[12] In a mouse tail model of psoriasis, *chi shao* promoted the growth of the granular layer in the mouse tail epidermis.[13]

Experimental Studies of *dan shen*

Lipid-soluble compounds of *dan shen* include tanshinone (I, IIA, IIB), iso-tanshinone (I, II), cryptotanshinone and dihydrotanshinone I, and the water-soluble compounds include salvianic acid and rosmarinic acid.[14–18] Experimental studies on *dan shen* have reported anti-inflammatory and antiproliferative effects.[2,4]

Salvianic acid A decreased intercellular adhesion molecule 1 expression in peripheral blood mononuclear cells extracted from a psoriasis patient.[19] Addition of tanshinone IIA to murine macrophages (RAW 264.7 cells) treated with LPS inhibited NF-κB, MAPKs (activator of 90-kDa heat shock protein ATPase homologue 1), ERK1/2 and JNK, as well as NIK (NF-κB-inducing kinase) and IKKα/β (IκBα kinase α/β).[20] In a similar model, a lipid-soluble extract of the *dan shen* root dose- and time-dependently inhibited NO production without cyto-toxicity, dose-dependently inhibited the mRNA and protein expression of iNOS, the levels of the pro-inflammatory cytokines TNF-α, IL-1b and IL-6 and intracellular ROS. It also significantly inhibited IκB-α degradation, NF-kB (p65) translocation, and CD14 (cluster of differentiation 14) expression. The authors concluded that the extract suppressed inflammation through NF-κB regulation.[21]

An aqueous extract of *dan shen* promoted the growth of the granular layer in the mouse tail epidermis which indicated a potential antipsoriatic effect.[13] Tanshinone IIA (Tan IIA) dose- and time-dependently inhibited the growth of keratinocytes and dose-dependently inhibited colony number growth curves. Apoptosis in cells treated with Tan IIA increased in a dose-dependent manner and caspase-3 and PARP increased in a dose-dependent manner in Tan IIA-treated cells. The authors concluded that Tan IIA inhibited the growth of keratinocytes via a caspase-dependent apoptotic pathway.[22]

Tan IIA concentration- and time-dependently decreased mitochondrial membrane potential and increased cytochrome c content. In a time-dependent manner, Tan IIA increased S and G2/M phase cells and decreased G1 phase cells. It also down-regulated cyclin A and pCDK2 (phospho-Cyclin-Dependent Kinase 2), which is associated with the S phase of the cell cycle, and down-regulated expression of PCNA which is involved in cell proliferation. Therefore, Tan IIA suppressed the keratinocytes via cell cycle arrest.[22]

Experimental Studies of *tu fu ling*

Tu fu ling has been reported to have antitumor and anti-inflammatory effects.[2,23] In a picryl chloride-induced contact dermatitis in mouse ears, pre-treatment with oral *tu fu ling* (100 mg/kg) inhibited the contact dermatitis. In a xylene-induced mouse ear model of inflammation, *tu fu ling* extract orally administered before the challenge, showed a trend towards inhibition.[24]

In a dinitrochlorobenzene-induced delayed-type hypersensitivity (DTH) mouse model of immune response, smiglabrin (a compound contained in *tu fu ling*) inhibited DTH, increased serum hemolysin and hemolytic plaque formation, and improved the phagocytosis of abdominal macrophages.[25]

Tu fu ling promoted the growth of the granular layer in the mouse tail epidermis which indicated a potential antipsoriatic effect. Also, *tu fu ling* significantly decreased endothelin-1 in mouse serum to a degree equivalent to methotrexate.[13]

Experimental Studies of *mu dan pi*

The *Paeony suffruticosa* root bark (*mu dan pi*) has been reported to have immune suppressive, anti-inflammatory and antiallergic actions.[3] It is one of the herbs that inhibits mitosis and PCNA expression in a mouse vaginal epithelium model, and promotes the growth of the granular layer in the mouse tail epidermis model of psoriasis.[13] It has also shown a significant inhibitory effect on human HaCaT keratinocyte cells *in vitro*.[26]

In primary normal human dermal fibroblasts and HaCaT cell lines, *mu dan pi* extract increased cell viability in these cell lines in a dose-dependent manner. Following fractionation, the effects were found to be related to the polyphenol fractions of condensed and hydrolysable tannins.[27] These studies suggest that *mu dan pi* has antiproliferative and wound-healing effects.

Experimental Studies of *bai xian pi*

Bai xian pi contains fraxinellone and dictamnoside A[28] and has been reported to have anti-inflammatory effects.[4,29]

An ethanol extract of the *bai xian pi* root bark dose-dependently inhibited histamine release from peritoneal mast cells and inhibited scratching behaviour in a mouse model of pruritus induced by compound 48/80.[30]

In mouse macrophage RAW 264.7 cells stimulated by LPS to produce an inflammatory response, pre-treatment with fraxinellone inhibited NO and PGE2 production and dose-dependently reduced the expression of iNOS and COX-2 which was due to the inhibition of NF-κB.[31] This suggests that this compound which is found in *bai xian pi* had anti-inflammatory effects.

In a mouse ear model of contact dermatitis induced by 1-fluoro-2,4-dinitrofluorobenzene (DNFB), topical application of a methanol extract of the *bai xian pi* root bark inhibited increase in ear thickness and weight and inhibited hyperplagia, oedema and spongiosis. The mice treated with the extract showed lower increases in IFN-γ and TNF-α levels in response to the DNFB challenge.[32] In a mouse tail model, *bai xian pi* promoted the growth of the granular layer in the epidermis indicating a potential anti-psoriatic effect.[13]

Experimental Studies of *zi cao*

Zi cao is mainly derived from *Lithospermum erythrorhizon* or *Arnebia euchroma*, though *Arnebia guttata* and *Onosma hookeri* can also be used. Each of these species contains shikonin and other compounds such as alkannin.[33] *Zi cao* has received considerable research attention for effects on inflammation, pruritus, proliferation, angiogenesis, wound healing and skin protection.[2,34]

In a passive cutaneous anaphylaxis (PCA) induced by DNP-HAS injection in rats, prior oral administration of a *zi cao* extract significantly inhibited PCA reaction. In murine peritoneal mast cells, the extract dose-dependently reduced compound 48/80-induced histamine release and in human mast cells (HMC-1), the extract reduced the production of the inflammatory cytokines IL-6, IL-8, TNF-α in response to phorbol myristate acetate plus A23187 stimulation. In addition, the extract inhibited the activation of the pro-inflammatory cytokine NF-κB by supressing IκB-α degradation.[35]

In an LPS-induced inflammation model in mouse macrophages, *L. erythrorhizon* extracts dose-dependently decreased levels of IFN-γ, TNF-α, IL-6, iNOS and IL-1β mRNA and suppressed the activation of AP-1 and NF-κB via suppression of IκB-α degradation.[36]

In an oxazolone-induced murine atopic dermatitis model, *L. erythrorhizon* extracts alleviated erythema, scaling and excoriation compared to the control. There was reduction in serum IgE, inhibition of COX-2 and iNOS, and attenuation of IkBα.[37] In an acute murine ear oedema model, the addition of topical shikonin dose-dependently reduced ear oedema by blocking the activation of IκB-α and thereby suppressing the activation of NF-κB.[38]

In a murine model of atopic dermatitis, an *L. erythrorhizon* root extract was administered to NC/Nga mice and found to reduce scratching behaviour in the experimental group. This was associated with lower serum IgE levels and an increase in epidermal ceramide level due to a reduction in ceramide degradation.[39]

An aqueous extract of *zi cao* had a strong inhibitory effect on vaginal epithelial cells and a linear dose-response was found for doses in the range 3.75 to 15 g/(kg·d).[40] In guinea pigs with epidermal hyper-proliferation induced by an essential fatty acid-deficient diet, oral dietary supplementation with *L. erythrorhizon* extract controlled the hyper-proliferation based on histological assessment and increased the ceramide level in epidermis.[41]

In human HaCaT keratinocytes that had been stimulated by IL-17, pre-treatment with shikonin dose dependently decreased VEGF mRNA expression vs. control, and also suppressed VEGF level in the supernatant vs. control. In human umbilical vein endothelial cells shikonin blocked VEGF-induced tube formation. In mice injected with recombinant mouse IL-17A into the ear, shikonin decreased VEGF and CD34 expression (dose dependently) vs. control.[42]

In a wound-healing model in rats, both shikonin and alkannin dose-dependently enhanced the proliferation of granulation tissue via increase in the number of CD11b+ cells in granulation tissue and accelerated proliferation of fibroblasts and collagen.[43]

Fractionated methanol extracts of *L. erythrorhizon* root were tested in human HaCaT keratinocytes to investigate the effects on serine palmitoyltransferase (SPT). Lithospermic acid and two derivative esters, 900-methyl lithospermate and 90-methyl lithospermate, raised the level of SPT protein in a dose-dependent manner, which suggests that these compounds could assist in recovery of normal epidermal permeability.[44] In cultured human keratinocytes and dermal fibroblasts an aqueous extract of *L. erythrorhizon* promoted wound healing at low doses by stimulating the movement, but not the proliferation, of both cell types and by accelerating lipid synthesis.[45]

These studies suggest that *zi cao* has anti-inflammatory, antipruritic, antiproliferative, pro-apoptotic, antiangiogenic and wound-healing effects.

Experimental Studies of *gan cao*

Gan cao (*Glycyrrhiza uralensis* root) has been reported to have immunosuppressive and immunoenhancing activities.[2] *Gan cao* compound glycyrrhetinic acid significantly inhibited the proliferation of RAW 264.7 macrophages stimulated by LPS.[46]

In human keratinocyte HaCaT cells, 10 to 100 μmol/L of glycyrrhetinic acid inhibited epidermal growth factor-induced cell proliferation in a dose-dependent manner. At 25 μmol/L, glycyrrhetinic acid inhibited epidermal growth factor-induced phosphorylation of ERK1/2, PCNA and Notch-1 expression.[47]

Experimental Studies of *ku shen*

The plant root contains more than 20 alkaloids, including matrine and oxymatrine, and a number of flavonoids.[48,49] *Ku shen* extracts and a number of its constituents have received research attention for their effects on inflammation and proliferation.[4,34,50]

Ku shen compound matrine demonstrated anti-inflammatory actions in HaCaT cells and in dermal fibroblasts which had been treated with substance P (SP). Matrine down-regulated production of IL-1β, IL-8 and monocyte chemotactic protein 1 in both cell lines.[51]

In a guinea pig model of psoriasis-like lesions, which had been induced by propranolol, the oral administration of matrine reduced ear thickness and decreased levels of IL-6, IL-8 and IL-17.[52] In a contact dermatitis mouse model in which ear swelling was induced by DNFB, the topical application of an extract of the *ku shen* root reduced hyperplasia, edema and spongiosis and suppressed increase in IFN-γ and TNF-α levels.[53] In RAW 264.7 cells, matrine, oxymatrine and sophordin inhibited CD91 and CD13 expression and inhibited the secretion of TNF-α.[54]

A prenylated chalcone (PC, 7,9,2',4'-tetrahydroxy-8-isopentenyl-5-methoxychalcone) isolated from *S. flavescens*, induced anti-inflammatory effects in HaCaT cells. It supressed Th2 chemokine expression, which had been induced by IFN-γ and TNF-α.[55]

An alkaloid-free prenylated flavonoid-enriched fraction derived from the *ku shen* root showed anti-inflammatory effects when applied orally in rats with adjuvant-induced arthritis. In a mouse macrophage-like cell line (RAW 264.7 cells) that had been treated with LPS to induce an inflammatory response, the *ku shen* fraction inhibited COX-2, iNOS and IL-6 with a lesser effect on TNF-α.[56]

In a psoriasis-like model which was induced by injection of IL-23 into mouse ears, topical kurarinone decreased ear swelling, reduced histological changes and inhibited the mRNA levels of IL-4, IL-17A and IL-22, inhibited the mRNA levels of inflammatory cytokines and chemokines related to psoriasis and inhibited the inflammatory mediators IL-1a, IL-1b, IL-6, TNF-α and COX-2. In addition, it increased mRNA levels of the anti-inflammatory cytokine IL-10. This suggests that kurarinone modulated cutaneous inflammation via the regulation of the CD4+ T-cell differentiation.[57] Trifolirhizin, a pterocarpan flavonoid extracted from *S. flavescens* roots, reduced LPS-stimulated inflammatory effects in mouse J774A.1 macrophages by reducing the expression of TNF-α, IL-6 and COX-2.[58]

In a mouse tail model, application of creams containing matrine at doses of 300, 200 and 100 mg/kg all showed promoting effects on the growth of the granular layer of mouse tail scale epidermis without producing side effects.[54] Oxymatrine showed inhibitory effects on mouse vaginal epithelial cell mitosis, reduced PCNA expression and decreased serum levels of IL-2, TNF-α and NO and increased IL-10.[59–61]

In a screen of herbs for antipruritic effects using mice with serotonin-induced itch, methanol extract of *ku shen* reduced scratching behaviour in a dose-dependent manner without producing sedation.[62]

These *in vitro* and *in vivo* studies indicate that compounds contained in *ku shen* can have anti-inflammatory, antiproliferative and antipruritic actions in models of relevance to psoriasis.

Experimental Studies of *di fu zi*

Di fu zi has been reported to have actions on inflammation, pruritus and proliferation.[29,63] An ethanol extract of the *Kochia scoparia* fruit and the oleanolic acid oligoglycoside, momordin Ic was found to have antipruritic activity and in subsequent *in vivo* experiments, momordin Ic had an antinociceptive in acetic acid-induced writhing and in a formalin test in mice. In rats, the extract reduced paw oedema that was induced by carrageenan.[64]

In a Freund's complete adjuvant reagent induced rheumatoid arthritis model in rats, momordin Ic and oleanolic acid showed anti-oedema effects and a similar result was found in a carrageenin-induced rat paw edema model.[65] In HaCaT cells and human fibroblasts (Hs-68), an ethanol extract of the *di fu zi* seed showed antiproliferative effects.[26]

These studies indicate *di fu zi* can reduce inflammation, pruritus and proliferation.

Summary of Pharmacological Actions of the Common Herbs

Herbs and their constituent compounds appear to have significant and concrete impact on reducing inflammation and proliferation. Each of the 11 herbs has evidently shown anti-inflammatory effects. Evidence for antiproliferative effects were also found in nine of the 11 herbs except for *zi cao* and *gan cao*. Other than these two major effects, the wound-healing function of *dang gui*, *mu dan pi* and *zi cao* may also play an important role in the treatment of psoriasis vulgaris. Furthermore, *zi cao*, *ku shen* and *di fu zi* have been proven to have antipruritic actions, which is beneficial for the main symptom of psoriasis vulgaris.

References

1. Zeng Y, Jia ZP, Zhang RX. (2006) 地黄化学成分及药理研究进展 [in Chinese]. *Chin Tradit Pat Med* **28**(4): 609–611.
2. Tse TW. (2003) Use of common Chinese herbs in the treatment of psoriasis. *Clin Exp Dermatol* **28**: 469–475.
3. Tan YQ, Liu JL, Bai YP, Zhang LX. (2011) Literature research of Chinese medicine recipes for the treatment of psoriasis vulgaris with blood-heat syndrome type. *Chin J Integr Med* **17**(2): 150–153.
4. Deng S, May BH, Zhang AL, Lu C, Xue CC. (2014) Phytotherapy in the management of psoriasis: A review of the efficacy and safety of oral

interventions and the pharmacological actions of the main plants. *Arch Dermatol Res* **306**(3): 211–229.

5. Baek GH, Jang YS, Jeong SI, Cha J, Joo M, Shin SW, Ha KT, Jeong HS. (2012) *Rehmannia glutinosa* suppresses inflammatory responses elicited by advanced glycation end products. *Inflammation* **35**(4): 1232–1241.

6. Liu CL, Cheng L, Ko CH, Wong CW, Cheng WH, Cheung DW, Leung PC, Fung KP, Bik-San Lau C. (2012) Bioassay-guided isolation of anti-inflammatory components from the root of *Rehmannia glutinosa* and its underlying mechanism via inhibition of iNOS pathway. *J Ethnopharmacol* **143**(3): 867–875.

7. Kuang YW. (2009) 鲜地黄叶中梓醇的积累动态及其抗银屑病作用的研究 [in Chinese]. Thesis. Academy of Military Medical Sciences, Beijing, People's Republic of China.

8. Han C, Guo J. (2012) Antibacterial and anti-inflammatory activity of traditional Chinese herb pairs, angelica sinensis and sophora flavescens. *Inflammation* **35**(3): 913–919.

9. Jing HX, Sheng WX. (2006) 当归多糖对豚鼠银屑病样皮损中角质形成细胞凋亡的影响 [in Chinese]. *Med J Wuhan Univ* **3**: 377–380.

10. Jing HX, Sheng WX, Duan DJ. (2008) 当归多糖对豚鼠银屑病样皮损中PCNA 表达的影响 [in Chinese]. *Chin J* **22**(1): 11–13.

11. Lee SJ, Lee IS, Mar W. (2003) Inhibition of inducible nitric oxide synthase and cyclooxygenase-2 activity by 1,2,3,4,6-penta-O-galloyl-beta-D-glucose in murine macrophage cells. *Arch Pharm Res* **26**(10): 832–839.

12. Chen T, Guo ZP, Jiao XY, Jia RZ, Zhang YH, Li JY, Huang XL, Liu HJ. (2011) Peoniflorin suppresses tumor necrosis factor-α-induced chemokine production in human dermal microvascular endothelial cells by blocking nuclear factor-κB and ERK pathway. *Arch Dermatol Res* **303**: 351–360.

13. Liu XM. (2011) 20 种中药灌胃对小鼠上皮细胞增殖和表皮细胞分化及血浆内皮素-1的影响 [in Chinese:]. *Chin J Dermatol* **34**(4): 282–283.

14. Li CG, Sheng SJ, Pang EC, May B, Xue CC. (2009) HPLC profiles and biomarker contents of Australian-grown *Salvia miltiorrhiza* f. alba roots. *Chem Biodivers* **6**(7): 1077–1086.

15. Wang X, Morris-Natschke SL, Lee KH. (2007) New developments in the chemistry and biology of the bioactive constituents of *Dan shen*. *Med Res Rev* **27**(1): 133–148.

16. Wu H. (2008) Research on pharmacological function of *Salvia miltiorrhiza*. *Acta Acad Zhejiang Univ Tradit Chin Med* **32**(5): 694–695.

17. Zhang Y, Jiang P, Ye M, Kim SH, Jiang C, Lu J. (2012) Tanshinones: Sources, pharmacokinetics and anti-cancer activities. *Int J Mol Sci* **13**(10): 13621–13666.

18. Zhou L, Zuo Z, Chow MS. (2005) *Dan shen*: An overview of its chemistry, pharmacology, pharmacokinetics, and clinical use. *J Clin Pharmacol* **45**(12): 1345–1359.

19. Wu JH, Yang SY, Jin L, Yang CX, Wu WY, Qin WZ. (1998) 丹参素对银屑病患者外周血单个核细胞黏附分子表达的影响 [in Chinese]. **25**(1): 47–49.

20. Jang SI, Kim HJ, Kim YJ, Jeong SI, You YO. (2006) Tanshinone IIA inhibits LPS-induced NF-κB activation in RAW 264.7 cells: Possible involvement of the NIK-IKK, ERK1/2, p38 and JNK pathways. *Eur J Pharmacol* **542**(1–3): 1–7.

21. Li M, Zhang L, Cai RL, Gao Y, Qi Y. (2012) Lipid-soluble extracts from *Salvia miltiorrhiza* inhibit production of LPS-induced inflammatory mediators via NF-κ, kappaB modulation in RAW 264.7 cells and perform anti-inflammatory effects *in vivo*. *Phytother Res* **26**(8): 1195–1204.

22. Li FL, Xu R, Zeng QC, Li X, Chen J, Wang YF, Fan B, Geng L, Li B. (2012) Tanshinone IIA inhibits growth of keratinocytes through cell cycle arrest and apoptosis: Underlying treatment mechanism of psoriasis. *Evid Based Complement Alternat Med* doi: 10.1155/2012/927658.

23. Jiang SJ. (2010 菝葜属植物菝葜和土茯苓现代研究概况) [in Chinese]. *Chin J Intern Med* **5**(2): 191–194.

24. Xu Q, Wang R, Xu LH, Jiang JY. (1993) 土茯苓对细胞免疫和体液免疫的影响 [in Chinese]. *Cell Mol Immunol* **9**(1): 39–42.

25. Bai L, Wu LY, Lian J, Zhou CM, Zhang KJ. (2003) 赤土茯苓苷对正常小鼠免疫功能的影响. 新疆医科大学学报 [in Chinese]. *J Xinjiang Med Univ* **26**(6): 573–574.

26. Tse WP, Che CT, Liu K, Lin ZX. (2006) Evaluation of the anti-proliferative properties of selected psoriasis-treating Chinese medicines on cultured HaCaT cells. *J Ethnopharmacol* **108**(1): 133–141.

27. Wang R, Lechtenberg M, Sendker J, Petereit F, Deters A, Hensel A. (2013) Wound-healing plants from TCM: *In vitro* investigations on selected TCM plants and their influence on human dermal fibroblasts and keratinocytes. *Fitoterapia* **84**: 308–317.

28. Gao X, Zhao PH, Hu JF. (2011) Chemical constituents of plants from the genus *dictamnus*. *Chem Biodivers* **8**: 1234–1244.

29. Yu JJ, Zhang CS, Zhang AL, May B, Xue CC, Lu C. (2013) Add-on effect of Chinese herbal medicine bath to phototherapy for psoriasis vulgaris: A systematic review. *Evid Based Complement Alternat Med* doi: 10.1155/2013/673078

30 Jiang S, Nakano Y, Rahman MA, Yatsuzuka R, Kamei C. (2008) Effects of a *Dictamnus dasycarpus* T. extract on allergic models in mice. *Biosci Biotechnol Biochem* **72**(3): 660–665.

31. Kim JH, Park YM, Shin JS, Park SJ, Choi JH, Jung HJ, *et al.* (2009) Fraxinellone inhibits lipopolysaccharide-induced inducible nitric oxide synthase and cyclooxygenase-2 expression by negatively regulating nuclear factor-κ, kappa B in RAW 264.7 macrophages cells. *Biol Pharm Bull* **32**(6): 1062–1068.

32. Kim H, Kim M, Kim H, Lee GS, An WG, Cho SI. (2013) Anti-inflammatory activities of *Dictamnus dasycarpus* Turcz., root T bark on allergic contact dermatitis induced by dinitrofluorobenzene in mice. *J Ethnopharmacol* **149**(2): 471–477.

33. Huang ZS, Zhang M, Ma L, Gu LQ. (2000) A survey of chemical and pharmacological studies on *zi cao*. *Nat Prod Res Dev* **12**(1): 73–82.

34. Deng S, May BH, Zhang AL, Lu C, Xue CC. (2014) Topical herbal formulae in the management of psoriasis: Systematic review with meta-analysis of clinical studies and investigation of the pharmacological actions of the main herbs. *Phytother Res* **28**(4): 480–497.

35. Kim EK, Kim EY, Moon PD, Um JY, Kim HM, Lee HS, *et al.* (2007) *Lithospermi radix* extract inhibits histamine release and production of inflammatory cytokine in mast cells. *Biosci Biotechnol Biochem* **71**(12): 2886–2892.

36. Han KY, Kwon TH, Lee TH, Lee SJ, Kim SH, Kim J. (2008) Suppressive effects of *Lithospermum erythrorhizon* extracts on lipopolysaccharide-induced activation of AP-1 and NF-κB via mitogen-activated protein kinase pathways in mouse macrophage cells. *BMB Rep* **41**(4): 328–333.

37. Lee JH, Jung KM, Bae IH, Cho S, Seo DB, Lee SJ, *et al.* (2009) Anti-inflammatory and barrier protecting effect of *Lithospermum erythrorhizon* extracts in chronic oxazolone-induced murine atopic dermatitis. *J Dermatol Sci* **56**(1): 64–66.

38. Andujar I, Recio MC, Bacelli T, Giner RM, Rios JL. (2010) Shikonin reduces oedema induced by phorbol ester by interfering with IκBα degradation thus inhibiting translocation of NF-κB to the nucleus. *Br J Pharmacol* **160**(2): 376–388.

39. Kim J, Kim Y, Seo D, Kim S, Lee S, Cho Y. (2009) Oral supplementation of *Lithospermum erythrorhizon* prevents the development of atopic dermatitis with reducing ceramide degradation in the epidermis of NC/Nga mice. *Phytother Res* **23**(9): 1250–1256.
40. Liu MQ. (2003) 不同剂量紫草水提液对实验性鼠阴道上皮细胞过度增殖抑制作用的初步研究 [in Chinese]. *J Clin Dermatol* **3**(12): 714–715.
41. Kim J, Kim H, Jeong do H, Kim SH, Park SK, Cho Y. (2006) Comparative effect of gromwell (*Lithospermum erythrorhizon*) extract and borage oil on reversing epidermal hyperproliferation in guinea pigs. *Biosci Biotechnol Biochem* **70**(9): 2086–2095.
42. Xu Y, Xu X, Gao X, Chen H, Geng L. (2014) Shikonin suppresses IL-17-induced VEGF expression via blockage of JAK2/STAT3 pathway. *Int Immunopharmacol* **19**(2): 327–333.
43. Ozaki Y, Sakaguchi I, Tujimura M, Ikeda N, Nakayama M, Kato Y, Suzuki H, Satake M. (1998) Study of the accelerating effect of shikonin and alkannin on the proliferation of granulation tissue in rats. *Biol Pharm Bull* **21**(4): 366–370.
44. Thuong PT, Kang KW, Kim JK, Seo DB, Lee SJ, Kim SH, Oh WK. (2009) Lithospermic acid derivatives from *Lithospermum erythrorhizon* increased expression of serine palmitoyltransferase in human HaCaT cells. *Bioorg Med Chem Lett* **19**(6): 1815–1817.
45. Kim H, Kim J, Park J, Kim SH, Uchida Y, Holleran WM, *et al.* (2012) Water extract of gromwell (*Lithospermum erythrorhizon*) enhances migration of human keratinocytes and dermal fibroblasts with increased lipid synthesis in an *in vitro* wound scratch model. *Skin Pharmacol Physiol* **25**(2): 57–64.
46. Jin RF, Liu J, Zhang JX, Tian YH. (2011) 甘草次酸及其衍生物 TY501 对小鼠巨噬细胞 RAW264.7 增殖的影响 [in Chinese]. Drug Eval Res **34**(4): 255–257.
47. Xian F. (2013) 甘草次酸抑制表皮生长因子对 HaCaT 细胞促增殖作用的机制研究. [in Chinese]. Thesis. Zhejiang Chinese Medical University, Zhejiang, People's Republic of China.
48. Ding H, Wang R, Gao Y, Zhao Q. (1995) The recent development of pharmacological and pharmacokinetic on the ingredients of *Sophora flavescens* root. *Chin Med Res* **4**: 63–64.
49. Liu G, Dong J, Wang H, Hashi Y, Chen S. (2011) Characterization of alkaloids in *Sophora flavescens* Ait. by high-performance liquid chromatography-electrospray ionization tandem mass spectrometry. *J Pharm Biomed Anal* **54**(5): 1065–1072.

50. Jin Y, Zhang HW. (2004) 苦参碱及氧化苦参碱的抗纤维化作用研究进展. [in Chinese]. *Chin J Integr Tradit West Nephrol* **5**(8): 493–494.

51. Liu JY, Hu JH, Zhu QG, Li FQ, Wang J, Sun HJ. (2007) Effect of matrine on the expression of substance P receptor and inflammatory cytokines reduction in human skin keratinocytes and fibroblasts. *Int Immunopharmacol* **7**(6): 816–823.

52. Sun CB, Zhu QG, Liu JY, Liu YS, Shen KY. (2009) . 苦参碱对普萘洛尔所致豚鼠银屑病样皮损的实验研究. [in Chinese]. *Pharm J Chin People's Liberation Army* **25**(6): 476–478.

53. Kim H, Lee MR, Lee GS, An WG, Cho SI. (2012) Effect of *Sophora flavescens* Aiton extract on degranulation of mast cells and contact dermatitis induced by dinitrofluorobenzene in mice. *J Ethnopharmacol* **142**(1): 253–8.

54. Liu TH, Liu DF, Wang C. (2010) 苦参碱乳膏对银屑病动物模型的实验性治疗研究. [in Chinese]. *Med J Natl Def Forces Southwest China* **20**(7): 714–716.

55. Choi BM, Oh GS, Lee JW, Mok JY, Kim DK, Jeong SI, Jang SI. (2010) Prenylated chalcone from *Sophora flavescens* suppresses Th2 chemokine expression induced by cytokines via heme oxygenase-1 in human keratinocytes. *Arch Pharm Res* **33**(5): 753–760.

56. Jin JH, Kim JS, Kang SS, Son KH, Chang HW, Kim HP. (2010) Anti-inflammatory and anti-arthritic activity of total flavonoids of the roots of *Sophora flavescens*. *J Ethnopharmacol* **127**: 589–595.

57. Kim BH, Na KM, Oh I, Song IH, Lee YS, Shin J, Kim TY. (2013) Kurarinone regulates immune responses through regulation of the JAK2/STAT3 and TCR-mediated signaling pathways. *Biochem Pharmacol* **85**(8): 1134–1144.

58. Zhou H, Lutterodt H, Cheng Z, Yu LL. (2009) Anti-inflammatory and antiproliferative activities of trifolirhizin, a flavonoid from *Sophora flavescens* roots. *J Agric Food Chem* **57**: 4580–4585.

59. Zhou R, Shi HJ, Jin SJ. (2010) 氧化苦参碱对银屑病样小鼠模型氧化应激的拮抗作用. [in Chinese]. *J Ningxia Med Coll* **32**(4): 481–483.

60. Shi HJ, Zhou R, Jin SJ, Yang J, Zhang XM. (2010) 氧化苦参碱对银屑病小鼠模型血清中 IL－2、IL－10、TNF—a水平的影响 [in Chinese]. *West China J Pharm Sci* **25**(4): 418–420.

61. Shi HJ, Zhou R, Jin SJ, Yang J, Zhang XM. (2011) 氧化苦参碱对银屑病模型雌激素周期小鼠阴道上皮细胞增殖和凋亡的影响 [in Chinese]. *J Clin Dermatol* **40**(11): 669–672.

62. Yamaguchi-Miyamoto T, Kawasuji T, Kuraishi Y, Suzuki H. (2003) Antipruritic effects of *Sophora flavescens* on acute and chronic itch-related responses in mice. *Biol Pharm Bull* **26**(5): 722–724.

63. Sun H, Fang WS, Wang WZ, Hu C. (2006) Structure-activity relationships of oleanane- and ursane-type triterpenoids. *Bot Stud* **47**: 339–368.

64. Matsuda H, Dai Y, Ido Y, Ko S, Yoshikawa M, Kubo M. (1997) Studies on kochiae fructus III. Antinociceptive and anti inflammatory effects of 70% ethanol extract and its component, momordin Ic from dried fruits of *Kochia scoparia* L. *Biol Pharm Bull* **20**(10): 1086–1091.

65. Choi J, Lee KT, Jung H, Park HS, Park HJ. (2002) Anti-rheumatoid arthritis effect of the *Kochia scoparia* fruits and activity comparison of momordin Ic, its prosapogenin and sapogenin. *Arch Pharm Res* **25**(3): 336–342.

7

Clinical Evidence for Acupuncture and Related Therapies

Overview

Acupuncture therapies have been used to treat dermatological conditions, including psoriasis vulgaris. Many clinical studies have been conducted both in China and internationally. This chapter provides an assessment of the current evidence from these clinical trials. Extensive searches of nine electronic databases identified 528 citations, which were reviewed against rigorous inclusion criteria. Finally, six clinical studies of acupuncture therapies for psoriasis vulgaris were selected for further analysis and are presented in this chapter. Controlled trials were subject to systematic review to evaluate the efficacy and safety of acupuncture therapies for psoriasis vulgaris. Non-controlled studies were examined to identify the acupuncture therapies used and the safety profile of these therapies. It was found that there is limited evidence for acupuncture therapies in treating psoriasis vulgaris.

Acupuncture is part of a family of techniques which stimulate acupuncture points to correct imbalances of energy and restore health to the body. Methods of stimulating acupuncture points include:

• Manual acupuncture: Insertion of an acupuncture needle into acupuncture points
• Electro-acupuncture: Application of an electrical stimulus to acupuncture needles
• Acupressure: Application of pressure to acupuncture points

- Auricular acupuncture: acupuncture at the points located on the auricle, also called ear-acupuncture
- Moxibustion: Burning of an herb (usually artemesia vulgaris) close to or on the skin to induce a warming sensation.

Whilst many of these therapies have ancient origins, several have emerged as new techniques in the last century. This includes auricular acupuncture, and electro-acupuncture therapies.

Previous Systematic Reviews

A search of currently available electronic databases did not identify any systematic reviews of acupuncture and related therapies for the treatment of psoriasis vulgaris.

Identification of Clinical Studies

A search of databases in English and Chinese identified 659 citations, and duplicates accounted for 131 of these citations. A total of 287 full-text citations were screened, where 268 did not meet the inclusion criteria, and thirteen studies were identified of interventions not commonly practiced outside of China, but they will not be presented here (Figure 7.1). After exclusions, two randomised controlled trials (RCTs) (S268, S269) and four non-controlled studies (S270–S273) of acupuncture therapy were included, while CCTs were excluded (Figure 7.1). One study was conducted in Sweden, and the remainder were conducted in China. Evidence from the controlled trials was evaluated for efficacy and safety, with RCTs providing the evidence.

In total, 279 people participated in these studies (Table 7.1). The mean age of participants ranged from 27 to 48 years. Duration of treatment ranged from three weeks (S273) up to ten weeks (S272). Comparators in controlled trials included sham acupuncture (S268), pharmacotherapy (acitretin) (S269).

Clinical Evidence for Acupuncture and Related Therapies

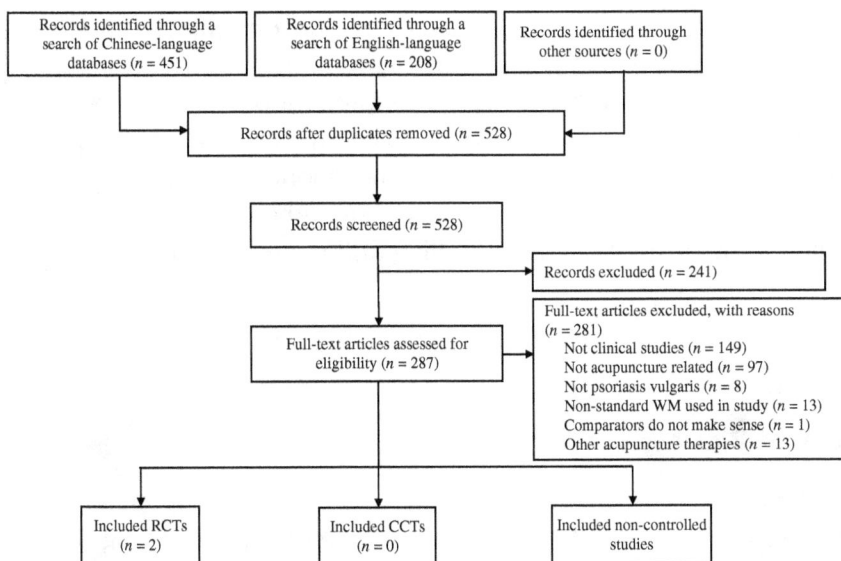

Figure 7.1. Flowchart of study selection process: Acupuncture and related therapies.

Table 7.1 Summary of Acupuncture and Related Therapies Clinical Studies

Study Design	No. of Studies	No. of Participants	Most Common Syndrome (No. of Studies)	Most Common Acupuncture Points (No. of Studies)
All clinical studies	6	279	Blood stasis and wind-dryness (3 studies) Blood heat (2 studies)	BL17 *Geshu* (5 studies) BL23 *Shenshu* (4 studies) SP10 *Xuehai* (4 studies) BL18 *Ganshu* (3 studies) LI11 *Quchi* (3 studies) LI4 *Hegu* (3 studies) SP6 *Sanyinjiao* (2 studies) ST36 *Zusanli* (2 studies) BL13 *Feishu* (2 studies) BL15 *Xinshu* (2 studies) GV14 *Dazhui* (2 studies)

Only three studies reported information on Chinese medicine syndromes (S270-S272). The most commonly reported syndromes included Blood stasis and wind-dryness and Blood heat. Interventions included acupuncture alone or in combination with moxibustion, and laser therapy. The most frequently reported acupuncture point was BL17 Geshu. Many of the most frequently used points have the function of clearing heat and cooling and moving Blood.

Randomised Controlled Trials of Acupuncture and Related Therapies

Risk of Bias Assessment

One RCT (S268) comparing acupuncture to sham acupuncture was assessed as 'low risk' for 'allocation concealment', 'blinding of participants', 'blinding of outcome assessors', and 'incomplete outcome data'; and 'unclear risk' for 'sequence generation', 'blinding of personnel' and 'selective reporting' due to lack of information. Another RCT (S269) comparing acupuncture plus moxibustion to acitretin was assessed as 'low risk' for 'sequence generation' and 'incomplete outcome data'; 'unclear risk' for 'allocation concealment', 'blinding of outcome assessors' and 'selective outcome reporting'; and 'high risk' for 'blinding of participants and personnel'.

Effects of Acupuncture

A single study involved 54 participants compared electro-acupuncture with sham acupuncture (S268), which found that electro-acupuncture was equally as effective as sham acupuncture for PASI score at the end of treatment and at follow up (MD 1.30 [–0.77, 3.37]). The study did not report on adverse events.

Effects of Acupuncture plus Moxibustion

One study compared acupuncture plus moxibustion with acitretin in 60 participants (S269). Results of PASI 95, 70 and 30 were reported, and for analysis, PASI 95 and 70 were combined under the outcome of PASI 60 or greater. Acupuncture plus moxibustion was equally as effective as acitretin in the number of people achieving PASI 60 (RR 1.31 [0.87, 1.97]). No adverse events were seen in participants who received acupuncture plus moxibustion, while those who received acitretin reported dry skin (10 participants), pruritus (seven participants), and desquamation (six participants).

Controlled Clinical Trials (Non-Randomised) of Acupuncture and Related Therapies

No CCTs of acupuncture and related therapies for psoriasis vulgaris were identified.

Non-Controlled Studies of Acupuncture and Related Therapies

Acupuncture therapies were described in four non-controlled studies (S270-S273). Interventions included acupuncture, and laser therapy. Five CM syndromes were reported, with Blood heat and Blood stasis with wind-dryness being reported in three studies each. The most frequent points were similar to those of all clinical studies.

Adverse events were reported by any of these studies.

Summary of Acupuncture Clinical Evidence

Results from single studies suggest that acupuncture plus moxibustion may be equally as effective as acitretin for the outcome PASI 60, and point application therapy may be equally as effective as halcinonide for lesion reduction and relapse rate. The disparate nature of the included interventions suggests that there is a lack of consistency in the clinical management of psoriasis in terms of acupuncture therapies used. However, there was some consistency across two studies in the acupuncture points suggested for use, whose actions reflect the suggested treatment principle for psoriasis.

These results should be interpreted with caution. The included studies all used different methods of point stimulation and different comparators, which did not permit pooling of results for meta-analysis. Further to this, differences existed in duration of disease, the sample sizes, duration of treatment and outcome measures, which may have contributed to the conflicting results.

Overall, there is limited evidence to support the use of acupuncture and related therapies for the treatment of psoriasis vulgaris, and no studies have evaluated their impact on health-related quality of life. Acupuncture in combination with moxibustion may be as effective as pharmacotherapy. Few clinical trials have been conducted, and well-designed clinical trials are needed.

When considering using acupuncture and related therapies for psoriasis vulgaris in clinical practice, points should be selected according to the point-specific function, and the syndrome of psoriasis shall be taken into consideration for selecting appropriate points. On the other hand, so far there is insufficient evidence to determine the safety of these therapies, and patients should be advised of the potential risk of Koebner phenomenon after treatment.

8

Clinical Evidence for Chinese Medicine Combination Therapy

Overview

In clinical practice, Chinese medicine therapies are often used in combination, such as Chinese herbal medicine plus acupuncture. Multiple studies have been published in scientific journals in China and internationally which have examined benefit of using Chinese medicine therapies in combination. Comprehensive search of nine databases identified few clinical studies, and when assessed against rigorous inclusion criteria only one randomised controlled trial was included in this chapter. In sum, there is limited evidence for the use of Chinese medicine therapies in combination for psoriasis vulgaris.

In clinical practice, Chinese medicine (CM) therapies are frequently used in combination to enhance the therapeutic effect. One randomised controlled trial (RCT) which combined CM therapies was identified from the electronic literature search.

Chinese Medicine Combination Therapy for Psoriasis Vulgaris

One study (S274) involving 66 participants used a combination of Chinese herbal medicine (CHM) bath and slide cupping applied to the lesion site. This was compared with NB-UVB and topical calcipotriol. The CM syndrome of Blood stasis was an inclusion criteria for the study. In terms of the methodological quality, this study was assessed as 'unclear' risk for 'sequence generation' and 'allocation concealment', 'high' risk for 'blinding of participants, personnel, and outcome assessors', 'low risk' for 'incomplete outcome data' and 'unclear' risk for 'selective reporting. The number of participants who achieved PASI 60 was no different in the CHM bath plus slide cupping group compared with NB-UVB and topical calcipotriol. Similarly, there was no difference between groups in PASI score at the end of treatment. These results show that the CM combination therapy group was equally effective as the comparator for the treatment of psoriasis vulgaris.

Summary of Main Findings

The included RCT provided evidence of efficacy of using CHM bath in combination with slide cupping for the management of Blood stasis-type psoriasis vulgaris. However, the very small number of included studies limits the certainty of the results. The slide cupping used in this study was not seen in the clinical studies in previous sections. Whether this technique is practical for psoriasis skin lesions remains unclear.

9

Summary and Conclusion

Overview

Chinese medicine therapies are increasingly used to treat psoriasis vulgaris, and a significant number of clinical studies have been conducted. Current conventional therapies are effective for psoriasis symptoms but usually do not cure the disease and may cause unwanted side effects with long-term use. Therefore, Chinese medicine is of significant value. Findings from clinical evidence revealed promising benefit of oral and topical Chinese herbal medicine, while evidence is lacking for acupuncture therapies and other Chinese medicine therapies. This chapter provides a 'whole-evidence' analysis in investigating Chinese medicine for the management of psoriasis vulgaris.

Considering that 'psoriasis' (or *Yin xie bing* in the Chinese language) is a modern medical term, in the classical Chinese medicine literature, a diversity of terms could refer to this disorder. Our systematic analysis found that *Bai bi*, *She shi* and *Bi feng* which appeared in the Ming dynasty, were the terms that were most frequently and consistently used to describe psoriasis vulgaris. Therefore, the treatment of these three conditions were considered as the mostly likely treatment used in history for managing psoriasis vulgaris. Current clinical guidelines or textbooks/monographs have recommended a variety of Chinese medicine (CM) therapies including both oral and topical Chinese herbal medicine (CHM), acupuncture, auricular acupuncture, and cupping therapy. Clinical evidence has been found to support the use of oral CHM and topical CHM;

however, the evidences for acupuncture related therapies and other CM therapies are insufficient.

Chinese Herbal Medicine

Both oral and topical CHM therapies have been cited in all forms of evidence in the treatment of psoriasis vulgaris. Oral multi-ingredient CHM, topical CHM ointments and CHM baths have all been suggested in historical medical books for treating this disorder. Contemporary textbooks and guidelines have also recommended these methods. In addition, several manufactured modern-style CHM products are also recommended by the contemporary literature. However, such manufactured CHM products have not all been evaluated by clinical trials.

In the classical literature, the CM aetiology of *Bai bi*, *She shi* and *Bi feng* conditions were believed to be caused by external wind, with internal Blood dryness being the underlying factor; consequently, the CHM treatments focused on dispelling wind (e.g. *Fang feng tong sheng san*, *Sou feng shun qi wan*). In the contemporary literature, external wind is not an important factor of the aetiology of psoriasis vulgaris. In fact, the syndromes of psoriasis vulgaris are all related to Blood: Blood heat, Blood dryness and Blood stasis. Accordingly, the CHM formulae or herbs recommended by current practice guidelines/textbooks are more focused on cooling or nourishing Blood or removing Blood stasis. In clinical studies, CHM formulae targeting these three Blood syndromes are also the most commonly reported. Other syndromes such as toxic heat were also found, albeit with a lower frequency.

Some of the CHM traditional formulae recommended by current practice guidelines/textbooks have been investigated by clinical trials; however, the number of studies applying the recommended formulae is relatively small. In fact, many formulae used in clinical studies did not have standardised names but may be modified forms of traditional formulae. The most frequently used herbs reported by all clinical studies were calculated, and included: *sheng di huang, dang gui, chi shao, dan shen, tu fu ling, mu dan pi, bai xian pi, zi cao, gan cao, ku shen* and *di fu zi.* These herbs have been proven to have one or more of the following psoriasis-related functions in experimental evidence: anti-inflammatory, anti-proliferative, anti-pruritic and wound-healing functions.

Clinical evidence have demonstrated that both oral CHM and topical CHM are beneficial for psoriasis vulgaris, in terms of PASI 60 or lesion reduction of 60%, particularly when used as an add-on therapy to pharmacotherapy or phototherapy. The frequently used herbs of studies included in positive meta-analyses are consistent with those reported by all clinical studies. Clinical studies also found that both oral and topical CHM are generally safe for psoriasis vulgaris patients, and as an add-on therapy, they can reduce common adverse events (AEs) caused by pharmacotherapy or phototherapy.

Summary of CHM across Evidence Types

Many herbal formulae have been recommended in clinical guidelines and evaluated in clinical studies. Table 9.1 lists the herbal formulae recommended in Chapter 2, and formulae that have been evaluated in two or more clinical studies. Some of these formulae are recommended in the contemporary literature; efficacy has been evaluated in clinical studies. There are also some CHM formulae (single- or multi-herb) assessed which have not been recommended in the contemporary literature. As discussed above, the understanding of psoriasis vulgaris in the classical literature is different to that in current practice. Therefore, the formulae that appeared in the contemporary literature or frequently evaluated in clinical trials did not show in the classical literature, and on the other hand, the formulae frequently cited in the classical literature did not appear in the contemporary literature or clinical studies.

Acupuncture and Related Therapies

Acupuncture therapy have been cited in the contemporary literature and evaluated in clinical studies. Moxibustion has also been

Table 9.1   Summary of Formulae

Formula Name	Evidence in Contemporary Literature	Evidence In Clinical Studies			Evidence in Classical Literature (No. of Citations)
		RCTs (No. of Studies)	CCTs (No. of Studies)	Non-Controlled Studies (No. of Studies)	
Oral CHM					
Dang gui yin zi	Yes	1	0	1	0
Fu fang qing dai wan (jiao nang)	Yes	1	0	3	0
Gan cao (single herb)	Yes	0	0	0	0
Lei gong tang duo gan pian	Yes	1	0	0	0
Qing dai (single herb)	Yes	0	0	0	0
Si wu tang	Yes	0	0	1	0
Tao hong si wu tang	Yes	1	0	5	0
Xiao feng san he xi jiao di huang tang	Yes	0	0	0	0
Xiao yin ke li	Yes	5	1	0	0
Huo xue san yu tang	No	2	0	1	0
Liang xue huo xue fu fang	No	2	0	1	0
Liang huo xue tang	No	2	0	0	0
Pi min xiao jiao nang	No	2	0	0	0
Run zao zhi yang jiao nang	No	3	0	0	0
Yang xue jie du tang	No	2	0	0	0

Topical CHM

Liu huang ointment	Yes	0	0	0	0
Bing hang fu le ointment	Yes	0	0	1	0
Pu lian ointment	Yes	0	0	0	0
Shi du gao	Yes	0	0	1	0
Qing dai gao	Yes	0	0	0	0
Qing dai ma you	Yes	0	0	0	0
Di yin xi ji	No	2	0	0	0

examined in clinical studies. However, the historical use of acupuncture and moxibustion therapies is uncertain.

Many of the clinical studies reported the CM syndromes seen in participants. Overlaps existed with the syndromes described in the contemporary literature. In addition, several clinical studies reported wind-heat, wind-dryness and internal toxic heat.

The most frequently reported acupuncture point was BL17 *Geshu*, reported in 83.3% of included clinical studies, where it has also been recommended by contemporary literature. Other frequently reported points were BL23 *Shenshu*, SP10 *Xuehai*, LI11 *Quchi*, and LI4 *Hegu*, each reported in 50% of included studies. Although these points were suggested maybe effective in contemporary literature, there was no supporting evidence in classical literature.

There is insufficient evidence from clinical studies to conclude on the efficacy and safety of acupuncture and related therapies for the treatment of psoriasis vulgaris.

Summary of Acupuncture and Related Therapies across Evidence Types

The nature of acupuncture practice has changed over time, and this is reflected in the number of citations, studies and recommendations for different therapies. The acupuncture therapies which have been recommended in contemporary literature, and therapies that have been evaluated in two or more clinical studies are listed in Table 9.2. There was no acupuncture related therapies recommended in classical literature. Among the acupuncture related therapies recommended by contemporary literature, acupuncture therapy has been evaluated by clinical studies, but not for auricular acupuncture.

Implications for Practice

International adoption and emphasis on evidence-based practice means that the future of CM will rely on clinical research to verify evidence from the classical literature and clinical practice. CM treatments should be considered in the context of medicine

Table 9.2   Summary of Acupuncture Therapies

		Evidence In Clinical Studies			
Acupuncture Therapy	Evidence In Contemporary Literature	RCTs (No. of Studies)	CCTs (No. of Studies)	Non-Controlled Studies (No. of Studies)	Evidence in Contemporary Literature
Body acupuncture	Yes	1	0	5	0
Auricular acupuncture	Yes	0	0	0	0

as a whole. With new information, we are better able to understand how, and to what extent, treatments improve specific aspects of psoriasis vulgaris. In fact, the research provides evidence which supports the recommendation for use of CM therapies, as well as validating new CM therapies, and highlights the importance of CM as one element in the overall care of psoriasis vulgaris patients.

Psoriasis vulgaris conditions were most likely to be *Bai bi, Bi feng* and *She shi* according to research of the classical literature. These terms first appeared in the Ming dynasty. The chief aetiology of such conditions were considered to be external wind invasion, and therefore the CHM treatment used in that period focused on expelling wind. Some traditional treatments are still used in current clinical practice. For example, CHM baths using herbs with functions of reducing itch or nourishing skin was cited in the classical literature, modern contemporary literature and clinical studies. Clinicians looking to the classical literature for guidance on selection of formulae should focus on those published in the Ming or subsequent dynasties with the terms *Bai bi, Bi feng* and *She shi*.

Research on herbal medicine toxicity has identified herbs which have toxic effects, such as *wu tou, ban mao, qian dan* and *shui yin,* which were cited in the classical literature. Since the discovery of toxicity, these herbs have not been recommended for skin conditions in clinical practice. Selection of herbs and formulae from the classical literature should be made in consultation with research on drug toxicity.

Findings from reviews of clinical evidence suggest CHM could be incorporated into an overall healthcare plan for psoriasis vulgaris. CHM formulae in clinical studies were selected or modified according to syndrome differentiation, which reflects clinical practice. This makes the evidence translatable to the clinical setting. Further, selection of formulae and herbs with consideration of concomitant pharmacotherapy allows clinicians to provide an effective treatment that may also reduce the side effects of medication.

Although acupuncture and related therapies are recommended in current CM clinical guidelines and textbooks, there is insufficient evidence to support the inclusion of acupuncture and related therapies as part of a healthcare plan for psoriasis vulgaris. There is little evidence to describe the safety of these interventions. As several acupuncture therapies involve skin penetration, and thereby adverse events such as micro-trauma and Koebner phenomenon may result from treatment. Patients should be advised of the potential risk of Koebner phenomenon prior to commencing treatment with acupuncture and related therapies.

Current CM clinical guidelines and textbooks do not recommend the use of other CM therapies, and few clinical studies have evaluated their benefit. The use of these therapies for the treatment of psoriasis vulgaris should be applied with caution.

Implications for Research

CM therapies are increasingly evaluated in clinical trials, in line with the development of conventional medicine. Our systematic analysis found that the current CHM managements of psoriasis vulgaris are consistent and encouraging; however, more evidence is needed for acupuncture therapies, especially as they are recommended in CM clinical practice guidelines. Further evidence is needed which addresses the following issues:

Methods

- Randomised controlled trials (RCTs) should be designed with rigorous methodology, with particular attention paid to adequate power and appropriate sample size calculation.
- Clinical trial protocols should be registered in the Clinical Trial Registry or be published prior to the conduct of RCTs to increase transparency in reporting.
- Outcome measures of psoriasis vulgaris should be validated and consistent with those recommended by international guidelines. Health-Related Quality of Life (HRQoL) measurement should be included as an important component in addition to symptom reduction.
- Considering that psoriasis vulgaris is a recurrent disease, the long-term effect of CM therapies for psoriasis vulgaris should be evaluated in follow-up phase using well validated outcome measures.

Intervention

- Researchers should explain the rationale for the use of intervention, including the dose and administration of CHM and the selection of acupuncture points.
- For CHM, authentication of raw material should be described and for manufactured products reports should include the quantity of active constituents.
- Syndrome differentiation should be considered in study design to improve applicability in clinical practice.

Reporting

- Research reports should follow the CONSORT statement with reference to the extension for herbal medicine[1] and STRICTA for clinical trials of acupuncture.[2]
- Individual modification of the prescription of CHM formulae or acupuncture points should be reported in more detail in order to instruct real-life clinical practice.

- Any modification or adjustment to the treatment method recommended by current clinical guidelines, and why and how, should be addressed when reporting the results.

Diversity was observed in the range of CM therapies, both within and across forms of evidence, reflecting the nature of CM clinical practice. Future research should focus on the most promising findings identified, and investigate therapies that can be widely used.

References

1. Begg C, Cho M, Eastwood S, Horton R, Moher D, Olkin I, Pitkin R, Rennie D, Schulz KF, Simel D, Stroup DF. (1996) Improving the quality of reporting of randomized controlled trials. The CONSORT statement. *J Am Med Assoc* **276**(8): 637–639.
2. MacPherson H1, White A, Cummings M, Jobst K, Rose K, Niemtzow R. (2001) Standards for reporting interventions in controlled trials of acupuncture: The STRICTA recommendations. *Complement Ther Med* **9**(4): 246–249.

Appendix 1: All Included Clinical Studies

Number	First Author, Year	Reference
S1	Ho SG, 2010	Ho SG, Yeung CK, Chan HH. Methotrexate versus traditional Chinese medicine in psoriasis: a randomized, placebo-controlled trial to determine efficacy, safety and quality of life. Clinical and experimental dermatology. 2010;35(7):717–22.
S2	Hu Liangpu, 2011	胡梁谱 and 胡静荣. 乌梅丸合麻杏薏甘汤加减治疗寻常型银屑病 50 例观察. 实用中医药杂志 2011;27(2):85.
S3	Li Shaohua, 2010	李芍华. 银屑敌治疗寻常型银屑病 30 例疗效观察. 哈尔滨医科大学学报. 2000;34(2).
S4	Li Yanxia, 2005	李炎夏. 阿维 A 联合中药消银方治疗寻常性银屑病疗效观察. 中国皮肤性病学杂志. 2005;19(4).
S5	Lin Mao, 2008	林茂, 熊芬, 侯秀芹, 熊心猜, 眭维耻. 乌梅合剂治疗寻常性银屑病临床观察. 医学信息(西安). 2008(1):111–2.
S6	Lin Rubin, 2009	林儒斌, 施银河, 钟来桂. 龙血竭胶囊治疗寻常型银屑病 60 例疗效观察. 赣南医学院学报. 2009;29(2):260.
S7	Lin Ruifeng, 2000	林瑞奋, 肖明辉, 王斗训. 三藤汤治疗寻常型银屑病临床及免疫学研究. 福建中医学院学报. 2000;10(3):8–10.
S8	Xu Ming, 2013	徐明. 清热凉血汤治疗寻常型银屑病血热证临床疗效观察. 辽宁中医药大学学报. 2013;15(1):177–8.
S9	Ma Xuewei, 2012	马学伟. 克银 I 号方对银屑病患者促细胞凋亡相关基因 Fas, bax 表达的影响. 中国老年学杂志. 2012;32(7):1385–1386.

(*Continued*)

(Continued)

Number	First Author, Year	Reference
S10	Ma Wanli, 2010	马万里, 曲永彬, 潘慧宜, 蒋淑明. 银屑病方治疗寻常型银屑病血热证 52 例疗效观察. 新中医. 2010(11):68–70.
S11	Ma Xuewei, 2011	马学伟, 陈虎, 张培红, 云雅卿, 王家颖. 克银i号方对寻常型银屑病患者血清白细胞介素-2、白细胞介素-2受体及肿瘤坏死因子-α 的影响. 河北中医. 2011;33(11):1617–9.
S12	Sun Jie, 2010	孙捷, 张虹亚, 刘小平. 复方泽漆冲剂对进行期寻常型银屑病患者生活质量的影响. 安徽中医学院学报. 2010;29(6):30–3.
S13	Tan Xinyun, 2008	谭新云, 刘慧文. 136 例寻常型银屑病的中西医治疗比较. 中外医疗. 2008;27(12):57–8.
S14	Wang Zhichun, 2003	王之春. 复方青黛胶囊治疗银屑病的随机双盲研究. 中国民间疗法. 2003;11(1):48–9.
S15	Wang Wenxing, 2012	汪文星, 汪洋. 香橼汤治疗寻常型银屑病临床观察. 湖北中医杂志. 2012(01):41–2.
S16	Xie Shaoqiong, 2009	谢韶琼, 易雪梅, 杨连娟, 李月萍. 抗银 1 号方治疗寻常型银屑病41例疗效观察. 河北中医. 2009;31(2):173–5.
S17	Xie Yong, 2006	谢勇. 退银汤联合阿维 a 胶囊治疗寻常型银屑病疗效分析. 实用中医药杂志. 2006;22(11):684–5.
S18	Su Xiaoyuan, 2010	苏晓媛, 王金海, 王峰, 郭强. 克银合剂治疗进展期血瘀型轻、中度寻常型银屑病疗效观察及对外周血 tnf-α, Tgf-β 水平的影响. 福建中医药. 2010;41(2):12–3.
S19	Yin Lihua, 2010	印利华, 常洪, 张永红. 清热凉血汤治疗寻常性银屑病 162 例疗效观察. 中国医学文摘(皮肤科学). 2010(05):282–3.
S20	Zhang Furen, 1999	张福仁, 田仁明, 马世尧, 汪新义, 于美玲, 施仲香. 雷公藤治疗进行期寻常型银屑病的随机双盲研究. 临床皮肤科杂志. 1999;28(1):32–3.
S21	Zhang Min, 2007	张敏, 张谊芝 and 汪盛. 阿维 A 治疗斑块状银屑病临床疗效观察. 临床皮肤科杂志. 2007;36(9):592–3.

(Continued)

(Continued)

Number	First Author, Year	Reference
S22	Zhou Meijuan, 2012	周梅娟, 王华, 黄艳, 崔丽萍, 陈云, 苗琦, *et al.* 凉血活血复方治疗进展期银屑病疗效及安全性评价. 中国中西医结合皮肤性病学杂志. 2012;11(3):152–4.
S23	Zou Jiyang, 2011	邹积阳. 消银颗粒治疗寻常型银屑病的应用研究. 中外健康文摘. 2011;08(29):110–1.
S24	Baoer Chulu, 2006	宝尔础鲁. 中西药结合治疗寻常性银屑病 96 例临床观察. 中国中西医结合皮肤性病学杂志. 2006;5(4):53.
S25	Cao Yuping, 2010	曹玉平, 李波, 王瑛. 自拟痒疹汤联合阿维 a 胶囊治疗寻常型银屑病疗效分析. 中国误诊学杂志. 2010(7):1553–4.
S26	Chen Bin, 2007	陈斌. 消银颗粒联合阿维 a 胶囊治疗寻常型银屑病 74 例. 现代中医药. 2007;27(6):29–30.
S27	Han Xiuqin, 2012	韩秀琴, 于海燕. 自拟凉血解毒养阴汤加减治疗寻常型银屑病 66 例疗效观察. 中医药导报. 2012;18(10):53–4.
S28	He Yongxiang, 2008	贺永香, 刘学东, 吕丽红, 周瑞. 消银一号合地蒽酚软膏治疗寻常型银屑病 108 例疗效观察. 当代医学. 2008(10):137.
S29	Hua Lidian, 2010	华黎电, 樊建勇. 阿维 a 联合中药清银解毒汤治疗寻常型银屑病疗效观察. 中药材. 2010(6):1026–7.
S30	Huang Yongjing, 2007	黄咏菁. 阿维 A 胶囊联合银屑灵片治疗寻常性银屑病的临床观察. 中国皮肤性病学杂志. 2007;21(10):I0003–I0004.
S31	Huang Zhiqiang, 2012	黄志强. 雷公藤多苷片联合他扎罗汀治疗寻常型银屑病 58 例. 中国实验方剂学杂志. 2012;18(15):276–8.
S32	Jiang Qunqun, 2012	姜群群, 陈洪晓, 刘卫兵. 参地颗粒联合阿维 a 治疗血热型寻常型银屑病疗效观察. 亚太传统医药. 2012;8(8):57–8.
S33	Jin Li, 2009	金力, 马一兵, 姜燕生, 娄卫海. 卡泊三醇软膏联合口服中药治疗寻常性斑块状银屑病的临床疗效观察. 中国中西医结合皮肤性病学杂志. 2009;8(4):216–8.

(Continued)

(Continued)

Number	First Author, Year	Reference
S34	Li Yaling, 2009	李亚玲. 三蕊胶囊与中药内服治疗寻常型银屑病. 中国社区医师·综合版. 2009(10):110.
S35	Li Wenxue, 2005	李文雪, 张振伟, 苗莹. 消疕汤混合维胺脂胶囊治疗寻常型银屑病 80 例. 陕西中医. 2005;26(6):517–8.
S36	Li Wenxue, 2010	李文雪, 雷明君. 中西医结合治疗寻常型银屑病 45 例. 四川中医. 2010;28(7):101–2.
S37	Liu Huanran, 2007	刘焕强. 消疕方联合阿维 A 治疗寻常型银屑病疗效观察. 辽宁中医杂志. 2007;34(6):786–787.
S38	Liu Jian, 2011	刘建. 卡泊三醇与皮敏消联用治疗寻常型斑块状银屑病的临床分析. 亚太传统医药. 2011;7(8):52–3.
S39	Liu Jinmin, 2012	刘津民, 刘英权, 李建英, 张玉红. 阿维 a 联合润燥止痒胶囊治疗寻常性银屑病临床观察. 中国中西医结合皮肤性病学杂志. 2012;11(1):32–3.
S40	Lu Yanshun, 2011	卢彦顺. 清凉解毒汤联合阿维 a 酯治疗银屑病临床研究. 中医学报. 2011;26(8):1001–2.
S41	Luo Changran, 2010	罗畅然, 马丽萍. 卡泊三醇联合皮敏消胶囊治疗寻常性斑块状银屑病疗效观察. 现代医院. 2010;10(7):44–6.
S42	Ma Shaoyun, 2012	马绍云, 徐晓燕. 阿维 a 胶囊联合大黄䗪虫丸治疗寻常性斑块状银屑病临床研究. 中国中西医结合皮肤性病学杂志. 2012;11(3):171–2.
S43	Meng Jun, 2004	孟军. 阿维 A 联合中药汤剂治疗寻常性银屑病临床观察. 中国中西医结合皮肤性病学杂志. 2004;3(4).
S44	Ou Bosheng, 2010	欧柏生, 冯杲. 中西医结合治疗寻常型斑块状银屑病疗效观察. 辽宁中医药大学学报. 2010(10):152–3.
S45	Tu Fuhan, 2011	屠福汉, 梁永妃, 施鉴勇. 润燥止痒胶囊治疗寻常型银屑病疗效观察. 浙江中西医结合杂志. 2011;21(7):489–90.
S46	Wang Wanchun, 2008	王万春, 熊佳玫, 马文军, 严张仁, 胡蓉, 封俊光. 中药联合甲氨蝶呤治疗寻常型银屑病 30 例疗效观察. 辽宁中医杂志. 2008;35(5):736–7.
S47	Xie Bo, 2012	谢波. 阿维 a 联合润燥止痒胶囊治疗寻常型银屑病的疗效观察. 中国医药指南. 2012;10(36):499.

(Continued)

(Continued)

Number	First Author, Year	Reference
S48	Xuie Yong, 2006	谢勇. 退银汤联合阿维 a 胶囊治疗寻常型银屑病疗效分析. 实用中医药杂志. 2006;22(11):684–5.
S49	Yu Qunce, 2008	于群策, 叶子. 清热凉血汤对寻常性银屑病患者 Th1/Th2 型细胞因子的影响. 中国中西医结合皮肤性病学杂志. 2008;7(3):155–7.
S50	Zeng Wenjun, 2009	曾文军, 王柳均. 复方丙酸氯倍他索软膏联合消银颗粒治疗寻常性银屑病疗效观察. 中国中西医结合皮肤性病学杂志. 2009;8(2):90–1.
S51	Zhai Xiufeng, 2012	窄秀凤. 阿维 A 联合中药治疗寻常型银屑病临床疗效观察 [硕士]: 天津医科大学; 2012.
S52	Zhang Zhenhan, 2012	张振汉. 中西医结合疗法治疗寻常型银屑病 56 例疗效观察. 中国医药指南. 2012;10(16):275–6.
S53	Zheng Xiaoyao, 2011	郑笑涛. 消银克疣汤治疗寻常型银屑病60例. 河南中医. 2011(04):383–4.
S54	Zhu Xiaoping, 2012	朱小平, 洪流. 中西医结合治疗寻常型银屑病的疗效分析. 四川中医. 2012;30(11):90–1.
S55	Zhu Hai, 2012	朱海, 邓景航, 黎晓琦. 中西医结合治疗寻常型银屑病的临床研究. 中国当代医药. 2012;19(35):104–5.
S56	Chen Ruiling, 2010	陈瑞玲. 化瘀消银汤联合紫外线治疗血瘀型银屑病疗效观察及对血流变影响的研究 [硕士]: 山东中医药大学; 2010.
S57	Cui Xin, 2005	崔欣. 窄谱中波紫外线及中药治疗寻常型银屑病的临床疗效观察 [硕士]: 南京中医药大学; 2005.
S58	Fu Shengxiang, 2007	伏圣祥, 王炜, 李明. 养血活血汤配合 nb-Uvb 治疗斑块状寻常型银屑病疗效观察. 中国麻风皮肤病杂志. 2007;23(9):824–5.
S59	Hao Sihui, 2006	郝思辉. 中草药煎服配合窄谱中波紫外线照射治疗寻常型银屑病疗效观察. 岭南皮肤性病科杂志. 2006;13(3).
S60	Huang Donghui, 2006	黄东辉. 火把花根片联合窄谱中波紫外线治疗寻常性银屑病疗效观察. 中国中西医结合皮肤性病学杂志. 2006;5(2).

(Continued)

(*Continued*)

Number	First Author, Year	Reference
S61	Liu YQ, 2011	刘屹球 and 严磊. 窄谱中波紫外线联合消银颗粒治疗银屑病临床观察. 临床皮肤科杂志. 2011;40(12):767–9.
S62	Lu Mao, 2009	陆茂, 叶俊儒, 张云光, 彭科, 沈跃莉. 窄谱中波紫外线联合中药治疗血燥型银屑病的疗效观察. 四川中医. 2009(12):102–3.
S63	Lv Huiqing, 2010	吕慧青, 郑玮清, 颜晓波. 凉血通络汤联合窄谱中波紫外线治疗寻常型银屑病临床观察. 中国中西医结合杂志. 2010(5):555–6.
S64	Lv Ping, 2009	吕萍. 克银丸联合 nb-Uvb 治疗寻常性银屑病疗效观察. 中国皮肤性病学杂志. 2009(8):539–40.
S65	Niu Runting, 2012	牛润亭. 窄波UVB联合凉血消风汤治疗血热型寻常型银屑病的临床和实验研究 [硕士]: 天津医科大学; 2012.
S66	Qin Jianwen, 2011	秦建文, 宋志刚. 窄谱中波紫外线照射联合复方鱼腥草软胶囊治疗寻常性银屑病临床观察. 中国民间疗法. 2011;19(12):47–8.
S67	Sun Wenyan, 2010	孙文眼, 阎慧军, 孔志凤, 赵莉. 化瘀白疕胶囊联合 nb-Uvb 治疗银屑病疗效观察. 光明中医. 2010(11):2013–4.
S68	Wang Guaijuan, 2008	王乖娟, 侯新江, 刘卫兵, 荆鲁华. 参地冲剂联合窄谱中波紫外线治疗血热型银屑病疗效观察. 中国中西医结合皮肤性病学杂志. 2008;7(2):98–9.
S69	Wang Guilin, 2010	王桂艳. 窄谱中波紫外线加中药治疗寻常性银屑病疗效观察. 中国中西医结合皮肤性病学杂志. 2010;9(3):168–9.
S70	Wang Linlin, 2006	王琳琳. NB-UVB 光疗治疗寻常型银屑病照射剂量、联合用药及作用机制的研究 [硕士]: 大连医科大学; 2006.
S71	Xie Xin, 2011	夏辛, 张文学. 凉血消风汤联合窄谱中波紫外线治疗寻常型银屑病疗效观察. 实用中医药杂志. 2011;27(6):371–2.
S72	Yan Huijun, 2011	阎慧军, 都群, 宋爱武. 乌蛇解毒丸联合窄波 uvb 治疗寻常性银屑病疗效观察. 中国社区医师·医学专业. 2011(2):127.

(*Continued*)

(Continued)

Number	First Author, Year	Reference
S73	Yu Lin, 2004	于霖. Goeckerman 疗法配合中药治疗银屑病临床疗效观察. 中国皮肤性病学杂志. 2004;18(1).
S74	Zhang Meiyu, 2008	张美玉, 李金立, 王东华. 凉血润燥汤配合窄谱中波紫外线治疗银屑病临床观察. 中国临床医生. 2008;36(1):55.
S75	Zhong, Jinbao, 2007	钟金宝. 窄谱中波紫外线联合"消银颗粒"治疗血虚风燥型银屑病 42 例. 岭南皮肤性病科杂志. 2007;14(2).
S76	Li Fei, 2009	李菲, 罗文辉. 中西医结合治疗寻常型银屑病 48 例. 湖南中医杂志. 2009(5):76–7.
S77	Liu Xuxing, 2005	刘旭星. 中药解毒凉血汤联合阿维 a 治疗寻常型银屑病疗效观察. 实用医技杂志. 2005;12(12A):3507–8.
S78	Wang Wuxing, 2012	汪五清, 高志祥, 郭志丽, 郭强, 杨勤萍, 顾军. 消银汤联合卡泊三醇软膏对血热型寻常性银屑病疗效及相关细胞因子水平的影响. 中华皮肤科杂志. 2012;45(9):647–9.
S79	Wei Guoxin, 2010	魏国信. 甘紫三七散治疗寻常型银屑病 100 例观察. 实用中医药杂志. 2010(11):755.
S80	Wu Shuidou, 2007	武水斗. 自拟消银汤加减治疗寻常型银屑病疗效观察. 中国误诊学杂志. 2007;7(13).
S81	Xu Ping, 2003	徐萍. 菝葜虎杖治银汤治疗寻常型银屑病临床研究. 国医论坛. 2003;18(3).
S82	Chen Guoquan, 2006	陈国权. 复方土茯苓汤联合阿维 A 治疗寻常性银屑病临床观察. 新疆中医药. 2006;24(1).
S83	Fan Min, 2003	樊敏. 小剂量维A酸联合消银肤乐饮治疗银屑病 150 例. 中国中西医结合杂志. 2003;23(10).
S84	Liao Lielan, 2009	廖烈兰. 阿维 a 联合中药治疗寻常型银屑病疗效观察. 中国麻风皮肤病杂志. 2009;25(2):143–4.
S85	Lv Yan, 2007	吕岩. 阿维 A 胶囊联合中药治疗寻常性银屑病疗效观察. 天津中医药. 2007;24(3).
S86	Shen Yunzhang, 2008	沈云章, 王景权, 徐新美. 雷公藤合剂治疗寻常型银屑病的疗效观察. 现代中西医结合杂志. 2008;17(23):3597–8.

(Continued)

(Continued)

Number	First Author, Year	Reference
S87	Xu Hao, 2011	徐皓, 唐红, 刘娟, 马玉宏. 清热凉血汤联合阿维 a 胶囊治疗寻常型银屑病 166 例. 陕西中医. 2011;32(6):706–7.
S88	Fan Wenhe, 2012	范文葛, 陶晓瑜, 王玲, 魏梅. 白芍总苷胶囊联合窄谱中波紫外线治疗寻常性银屑病. 中华皮肤科杂志. 2012;45(10):755–6.
S89	Gu Songjie, 2011	顾松杰, 桑振华. 消风颗粒联合窄谱中波紫外线照射治疗寻常型银屑病 42 例. 河南中医. 2011; 31(11):1310–1.
S90	Pan Shaoying, 2012	潘少英. 光疗联合消银颗粒治疗寻常性银屑病 26 例. 中国中医药现代远程教育. 2012(24).
S91	Yang Bo, 1980	杨波, 中医辨证论治治疗 20 例银屑病临床观察. 铁道医学. 1980(05):262–263.
S92	Xu Zongxian, 2003	徐宗贤, 蔡累 and 陆承光, 自制银消片治疗银屑病 200 例疗效观察. 中华新医学. 2003;4(16): 1522–1523.
S93	Xiong Bo, 2004	熊波, 从瘀论治稳定期银屑病 50 例. 湖北中医杂志. 2004;26(3):C29.
S94	Xie Suhua, 2009	谢素华, 中医治疗银屑病探索. 中国民族民间医药杂志. 2009;18(7):41–42
S95	Xiao Lichun, 2004	肖春丽, 中药内服外洗治疗银屑病 46 例小结. 湖南中医药导报. 2004, 10(6):42.
S96	Xian Xiaoli, 2002	线晓莉, 活血化淤法治疗银屑病 50 例观察. 黑龙江医药. 2002; 15(2):
S97	Xie Qingmei, 2007	夏庆梅, 凉血活血消银汤治疗寻常型银屑病 40 例. 天津中医药. 2007;24(1):54.
S98	Wu Juansheng, 2003	吴跃申, 周群, 徐琴言 and 水润英, 清热解毒汤治疗老年热毒型银屑病的疗效、安全性临床探讨. 2003;2003中国中西医结合皮肤性病学术会议.
S99	Wu Size, 1994	吴思泽, 复方青黛丸治疗银屑病 89 例疗效观察. 安徽医学. 1994;15(2):26.
S100	Wu Lihua, 2003	吴丽华, 中医辨症治疗银屑病 42 例临床疗效观察. 皮肤病与性病. 2003;25(4):30–31.

(Continued)

(Continued)

Number	First Author, Year	Reference
S101	Wei Lingjie, 2008	韦灵杰, 银消丸治疗白疕 627 例临床观察. 中国中医药现代远程教育. 2008;6(12):
S102	Wang Zhoukang, 2002	王宙康, 牛皮癣丸治疗银屑病 160 例. 2002 中国中西医结合皮肤性病学术会议. 2002.
S103	Wang Yuqi, 2011	王玉奇, 银屑 1 号治疗寻常型银屑病 92 例. 光明中医. 2011;26(7):1401.
S104	Wang Yajuan, 2003	王雅娟, 紫草活血汤治疗银屑病的疗效及对血液流变学的影响. 西安交通大学学报(医学版). 2003;24(3):C29.
S105	Wang Xiaobing, 2012	王晓兵, 中医辨证治疗寻常型银屑病 48 例临床观察. 内蒙古中医药. 2012;31(9):2.
S106	Wang Junhui, 2011	王俊慧, 刘瓦利, 闫雨荷, 何伟 and 王君伟, 清热凉血解毒法治疗寻常型银屑病血热证的重复测量分析. 辽宁中医杂志. 2011;38(1):29–31.
S107	Wang Huanchao, 1990	王桓朝, 皮炎汤治疗皮肤病验案. 北京中医. 1990; (03):4–5.
S108	Wang Feng, 2001	王峰 and 郭梅, 紫灵消银丸治疗银屑病 102 例. 2001 年中国中西医结合皮肤性病学术会议. 2001.
S109	Wang Dehui, 1987	王德慧, 雷公藤合剂配扶正祛邪中药治疗 36 例寻常型银屑病的临床观察. 南京中医学院学报. 1987; (01):11–12.
S110	Wang Wuqing, 2012	汪五清, 王峰, 高志祥, 卜晓琳 and 顾军, 消银汤对血热型银屑病患者疗效及外周血 T-bet/GATA3 平衡的影响. 中国中西医结合皮肤性病学杂志. 2012;11(2):74–77.
S111	Tao Guiyi, 1993	陶贵义, 清热利湿法治疗家族性银屑病 3 例. 黑龙江中医药. 1993;(1):28.
S112	Sun Zhong, 2004	孙忠, 驱风燥湿补肾理血法治疗寻常型银屑病 88 例临床观察. 中华中医药学会皮肤科分会学术会议. 2004.
S113	Sun Youqin, 1982	孙佑勤, 菝葜、土茯苓治疗银屑病 108 例疗效观察. 北镇医学院学报. 1982;(1):46–50.
S114	Sun Li, 1999	孙莉, 曹桂英 and 付香芹, 复方青黛胶囊治疗皮肤病的中医护理. 黑龙江中医药. 1999;(04):47.

(Continued)

(Continued)

Number	First Author, Year	Reference
S115	Sun Guoqiang, 2009	孙国强, 润燥凉血汤对寻常型银屑病患者血浆血管内皮生长因子含量的影响. 时珍国医国药. 2009;20(7):C29.
S116	Sun Benhai, 1997	孙本海, 卢庆芳 and 卢庆菊, 复方青黛胶囊治疗银屑病疗效观察. 岭南皮肤性病科杂志. 1997;4(3):40,23.
S117	Sun Baofang, 2008	孙保芳 and 张玉勇, 自拟"四逆石膏汤"治疗银屑病5o例疗效观察. 中外医疗. 2008;27(12):63.
S118	Song Guangying 1999	宋广英, 从"血"论治寻常型银屑病 56 例. 广西中医药. 1999;22(5):C29.
S119	Shi Zhichao, 1989	石志超 and 王勇, 乌蛇搜风汤治疗银屑病 64 例. 陕西中医. 1989;(02):64–65.
S120	Shi Chengyi, 2011	石成义, 分型辨证治疗寻常型银屑病 46 例疗效观察. 北京中医药. 2011;30(9):686–687.
S121	Shi Qingbao, 1998	施庆保, 复方青黛丸治疗银屑病 308 例疗效观察. 皮肤病与性病. 1998;20(2):30.
S122	Shen Zhongwen, 1987	沈仲文, 自拟中药"抗银丸"治疗寻常型银屑病 73 例临床观察. 贵阳中医学院学报. 1987;(3):28–29.
S123	Shen Yue, 1997	沈悦 and 汤效群, 凉血活血祛风解毒为主治疗银屑病 68 例. 南京中医药大学学报. 1997;(02):49–50.
S124	Shen Qingyi, 2008	沈庆毅, 自拟速效消斑散治疗银屑病 368 例. 云南中医中药杂志. 2008;29(11):39–40.
S125	Shen Jingnan, 1995	沈镜南 and 吴伊旋, 珍羚合剂口服液治疗热毒所致皮肤炎症. 中成药. 1995;17(12):23–24.
S126	Sang Xudong, 2011	桑旭东, 分期辨治寻常型银屑病 120 例. 山东中医药大学学报. 2011;35(1):41–43.
S127	Rong Xianhui, 2006	荣显会, 透疹解毒散治疗与感染相关的寻常性银屑病. 河北中医药学报. 2006;21(2):C29.
S128	Ren Xixiang, 2006	任锡祥, 通圣四物汤治疗寻常性银屑病 124 例临床观察. 中外健康文摘: 医药月刊. 2006;3(11):C29.
S129	Ren Haiping, 2008	任海平 and 任雁翔, 化瘀润肤消斑汤治疗寻常型银屑病 120 例. 实用中医药杂志. 2008;24(8):501.

(Continued)

(Continued)

Number	First Author, Year	Reference
S130	Ren Haiping, 2005	任海平, 化瘀润燥法治疗寻常型银屑病 120 例疗效观察. 中国临床医药研究杂志. 2005;(138): 14971–14972.
S131	Quan Zhijie, 1987	权志杰, 复方山豆根片治疗银屑病 50 例疗效观察. 兰后卫生. 1987;(1):33.
S132	Quan Yaoheng, 2008	权耀恒 and 权敬梓, 克银方治疗银屑病 93 例临床观察. 山东中医杂志. 2008;27(7):467–468.
S133	Qiu Ningcai, 1990	裘凝才, 中医分型治疗银屑病 681 例疗效观察. 北京中医. 1990;(4):19–20.
S134	Qiu Guirong, 2007	邱桂荣, 辨证论治配合小剂量雷公藤多甙治疗寻常型银屑病 184 例临床体会. 中华中医药学会皮肤科分会第四次学术年会. 2007.
S135	Qian Fei, 2006	钱斐, 自拟凉血解毒汤治疗血热型银屑病 76 例. 卫生职业教育. 2006;24(23):128.
S136	Pi Juchuan, 1995	皮巨川, 犀角地黄汤加味治疗寻常型银屑病 26 例疗效观察. 贵阳中医学院学报. 1995;17(1):57–58.
S137	Pei Wentao, 2009	裴文涛 and 王思农, 犀角地黄汤加减治疗寻常型银屑病 40 例. 甘肃中医. 2009;22(3):40–41.
S138	Pan Baohua, 1994	潘保华, 李彩萍, 贾蕴强, 郭明慧 and 朱达基, 北芪菇对银屑病疗效的初步研究. 食用菌. 1994; 16(5):43.
S139	Ma Shouze, 1993	马守泽, 中药全蝎黄酒治疗银屑病疗效观察. 中国皮肤性病学杂志. 1993;7(2):114.
S140	Ma Lin, 2005	马林, 凉血消银汤加减治疗寻常型银屑病 60 例. 中医研究. 2005;18(1):
S141	Lv Hekun, 2009	吕和坤, 银屑灵治疗银屑病 91 例. 现代中医药. 2009;(3):31.
S142	Lu Bin, 2004	路斌, 消银汤治疗寻常型银屑病 76 例. 四川中医. 2004;22(7):
S143	Lu Jun Fang, 2001	卢俊芳, 从血论治进行期银屑病 46 例疗效观察. 皮肤病与性病. 2001;23(2):
S144	Lou Yuanming, 1996	娄渊明, 自拟"莪术乌梅汤"治疗银屑病的临床观察. 中国农村医学. 1996;24(6):58.

(Continued)

(*Continued*)

Number	First Author, Year	Reference
S145	Liu Xiyu, 2009	柳锡余, 中医辨证治疗寻常型银屑病 60 例. 湖北中医杂志. 2009;31(9):64–65.
S146	Liu Zihang, 2010	刘子航, 中医辨证治疗寻常型银屑病疗效观察. 中国中医药咨讯. 2010;(7):189.
S147	Liu Yan, 1999	刘燕, 中医治疗银屑病 285 例疗效观察. 皮肤病与性病. 1999;21(4):
S148	Liu Xijuan, 1999	刘西娟 and 刘品莉, 凉血解毒汤加减治疗银屑病临床报道. 中医药研究. 1999;15(2):17–18.
S149	Liu Wenjing, 1997	刘文景, 凉血解毒汤治疗寻常型银屑病 106 例. 山东中医杂志. 1997;16(1):16–17.
S150	Liu Shigang, 1999	刘世刚 and 李建国, 土槐饮治疗银屑病. 山东中医杂志. 1999;18(12):547–548.
S151	Liu Peihong, 2005	刘培红, 凉血除银汤治疗寻常型进行期银屑病 68 例. 天津中医药. 2005;22(6):
S152	Liu Limin, 1999	刘利民, 李玉梅 and 王丽华, 银屑病 1 号冲剂的研制及126 例临床疗效观察. 黑龙江医药. 1999;12(6):370–371.
S153	Liu Lan, 2008	刘岚, "消疕汤"治疗寻常型银屑病 46 例. 江苏中医药. 2008;40(4):27.
S154	Liu Jian, 2011	刘建, 韩景智, 冯世军 and 赵丽, 清热凉血洗剂外敷治疗寻常型银屑病. 中医临床研究. 2011;3(20):42.
S155	Liu Huanqing, 2007	刘环清, 凉膈散加减治疗寻常型银屑病的临床观察. 中国中医药科技. 2007;14(4):234.
S156	Liu Cankun, 2006	刘灿坤 and 周评, 银屑口服液治疗寻常型银屑病疗效观察. 医药世界. 2006;(4):90–91
S157	Ling Xinmin, 1994	凌新民, 克银方治疗寻常型银屑病 72 例疗效观察. 光明中医. 1994;(1):25–27.
S158	Lin Hai, 2006	林海, 清肺透表祛湿解毒法治疗寻常型银屑病及血清 IL-8 水平检测. 中国中医急症. 2006;15(12):
S159	Liang Shangcai, 2005	梁尚财 and 许先斌, 试论寻常型银屑病中医治疗方法:附 50 例临床分析. 中华现代皮肤科学杂志. 2005;2(5):439–441.
S160	Liang Shangcai, 2005	梁尚财, 中医治疗寻常型银屑病 50 例. 吉林中医药. 2005;25(11):

(*Continued*)

(Continued)

Number	First Author, Year	Reference
S161	Liang Dequan, 2012	梁德权, 自拟凉血解毒汤治疗点滴状银屑病疗效观察. 医学理论与实践. 2012;25(10):1247.
S162	Liang Bingjun, 2010	梁秉钧, 自拟凉血地黄汤治疗寻常型银屑病 46 例. 中国社区医师·综合版. 2010;(17):131.
S163	Li Zongming, 2010	李宗民 and 孙晓莉, 中医辨证治疗寻常型银屑病 575 例疗效分析. 吉林中医药. 2010;30(8): 693–694.
S164	Li Zhuangyuan, 2008	李庄原, 银屑病的中医辨证治疗. 临床医药实践. 2008;17(8):693,718.
S165	Li Zhenlu, 2002	李振鲁, 消银化瘀汤治疗银屑病临床研究. 中国误诊学杂志. 2002;2(8):
S166	Li Yongmei, 2004	李咏梅, 马绍尧 and 宋瑜, 中医辨证治疗寻常型银屑病 450 例疗效观察. 中华现代中西医杂志. 2004;2(2):153–154.
S167	Li Yinglin, 2002	李映琳, 消银解毒方治疗银屑病 573 例. 北京中医药大学学报. 2002;25(6):
S168	Li Yinfang, 1997	李荫芳 and 李淑侠, 辨证分型治疗白疕病 110 例. 陕西中医学院学报. 1997;20(1):24–25.
S169	Li Taohua, 2010	李桃花 and 瞿幸, 银屑病中医证候演变规律及疗效观察. 北京中医药大学学报. 2010;(4):286–288.
S170	Li Shufen, 1988	李淑芬, 中药治疗银屑病 143 例临床观察. 吉林中医药. 1988;(4):17.
S171	Li Ming, 1994	李明 and 李玲, 通导散治疗银屑病 45 例. 山东中医杂志. 1994;13(7):300–301.
S172	Li Maoyu, 2012	李茂雨, 133 例银屑病的中医治疗. 中国保健营养（中旬刊）2012.
S173	Li Maoxing, 1993	李茂兴, 银屑病从"血"论治 376 例疗效观察. 河北中医. 1993;15(3):27–28.
S174	Li Hua, 2012	李华, 自拟消银汤治疗寻常型银屑病（血热证）疗效观察及对外周血 T 淋巴细胞亚群的影响. 成都中医药大学. 硕士. 2012.
S175	Li Fenghui, 1997	李凤辉, 中医辨证治疗银屑病 40 例临床疗效观察. 四川中医. 1997;15(9):44.

(Continued)

(Continued)

Number	First Author, Year	Reference
S176	Li Chao, 2004	李超, 一清胶囊治疗寻常型银屑病疗效观察. 工企医刊. 2004;17(5):57.
S177	Li Anhai, 2013	李安海, 辨证治疗寻常型银屑病 96 例. 山东中医杂志. 2013;(03):168–169.
S178	Leng Xueying, 2012	冷雪英, 驱风燥湿补肾理血法治疗寻常型银屑病 88 例临床观察. 中外健康文摘. 2012;(38):
S179	Lei Sanli, 2007	雷三礼 and 刘发利, 青黛薜皮汤治疗银屑病 54 例临床观察. 实用医技杂志. 2007;14(18):2474–2475.
S180	Le Qi, 2001	乐奇, 中药治疗进行期银屑病 56 例. 成都中医药大学学报. 2001;24(2):63.
S181	Kang Guozhi, 2006	康果枝, 消银凉血饮治疗银屑病90例疗效观察. 山西中医. 2006;22(4):25–26.
S182	Jin, Xiamin, 1997	荆夏敏, 谷淑梅 and 巩晓玲, 温阳活血化瘀汤治疗银屑病 100 例. 陕西中医. 1997;18(5):208.
S183	Jin, Qifeng, 1983	金起凤, 消银汤治疗银屑病 58 例疗效观察. 辽宁中医杂志. 1983;(6):29–30.
S184	Jiang Zhonghui, 2011	蒋中会, 解毒凉血汤治疗寻常型银屑病 30 例. 现代中医药. 2011;31(5):49–50.
S185	Jiang Xindao, 2005	姜新道, 自拟克银汤治疗血热型银屑病临床观察. 青岛医药卫生. 2005;37(4):
S186	Jiang Shikui, 2007	姜世奎, 活血补气法治疗老年性银屑病 58 例疗效观察. 中国实验方剂学杂志. 2007;13(6):
S187	Jia, Zhonghua, 1998	贾中华 and 桑智先, 银屑灵冲剂治疗寻常型银屑病. 山东中医杂志. 1998;17(3):111–112.
S188	Huang Zhonggui, 2002	黄仲贵, 四物汤加减治疗寻常型银屑病 18 例. 皮肤病与性病. 2002;24(3):
S189	Huang Ping, 2009	黄萍, 牛皮癣 II 号汤剂对血热型寻常型银屑病患者血清 mmp-2 及 mmp-9 水平的影响. 辽宁中医杂志. 2009;(5):786–787.
S190	Hua Gang, 2003	华刚, 辨证论治银屑病 78 例. 四川中医. 2003; 21(5): 61–62.
S191	Hu Yanjun, 2000	胡艳君, 凉血消银汤治疗进行期银屑病 58 例. 陕西中医. 2000;21(7):305.

(Continued)

(*Continued*)

Number	First Author, Year	Reference
S192	Hou Suchun, 2006	侯素春, 中药凉血活血复方治疗银屑病 133 例临床疗效观察. 临床皮肤科杂志. 2006;35(11):
S193	Hou Ming, 2008	侯明, 凉血解毒汤治疗银屑病临床疗效观察. 辽宁中医杂志. 2008;35(3):408–409.
S194	He Qin, 2012	贺勤, 白芍总苷对寻常型银屑病患者皮损 IL-17 表达的影响. 医药导报. 2012;31(7):
S195	Han Zhongcheng, 1989	韩仲成, 麻杏薏甘汤加味治疗银屑病临床观察. 山西中医. 1989;5(3):25–26.
S196	Han Shouzhang, 2001	韩首章, 自拟消银煎治疗寻常型银屑病 160 例. 辽宁中医杂志. 2001;28(10):
S197	Han Shirui, 2005	韩石蕊, 鲜苓消银胶囊的制备及疗效观察. 光明中医. 2005;20(2):
S198	Han Qingli, 1998	韩丽清, 扶正消毒饮治疗点滴型银屑病 36 例临床观察. 内蒙古中医药. 1998;17(4):16.
S199	Guo Jianhui, 2011	郭建辉, 郭雯 and 付红娟, 化瘀通络方治疗寻常型银屑病血瘀证疗效观察. 中医临床研究. 2011; 3(21):91.
S200	Gong Jinglin, 1996	龚景林, 消银饮治疗银屑病 100 例疗效观察. 湖南中医杂志. 1996;12(2):34.
S201	Gong He, 2004	龚合, 祖国医学治疗寻常型银屑病 157 例. 中华医学写作杂志. 2004;11(8):673–675.
S202	Gao Shaozuo, 1997	高绍佐, 雷公藤治疗银屑病疗效分析. 皮肤病与性病. 1997;19(4):26.
S203	Feng Jie, 1996	冯捷, 徐汉卿 and 苏宝山, 复方青黛胶囊对银屑病表皮角朊细胞中 c-Myc 表达的影响. 中国中西医结合杂志. 1996;16(3):146–148.
S204	Fan Xiaosan, 2011	范孝叁, 加味土槐饮治疗寻常型银屑病 72 例. 云南中医中药杂志. 2011;32(5):42.
S205	Duan Xiufeng, 2001	段秀峰, 双山克银片治疗银屑病 390 例. 吉林中医药. 2001;21(3):
S206	Du Xuemei, 2002	杜雪梅, 自拟凉血解毒汤治疗血热型银屑病 76 例. 辽宁中医学院学报. 2002;4(3):
S207	Du Fengwen, 2003	杜锋文, 自拟三藤汤治疗银屑病 100 例分析. 中医药学刊. 2003;21(10):

(*Continued*)

(*Continued*)

Number	First Author, Year	Reference
S208	Dong Yuchi, 2001	董玉池, 寻常型银屑病辩证治疗心得. 2001 年中国中西医结合皮肤性病学术会议. 2001.
S209	Donbg Yongfeng, 1987	董永丰, 银屑平治疗银屑病 460 例临床观察. 陕西中医. 1987;(12):535–536.
S210	Ding Wenling, 2002	丁文玲 and 李同银, 五福灵犀丹治愈点滴状银屑病 1 例. 中国民间疗法. 2002;10(12):45.
S211	Deng Jingwen, 2012	邓静文, 银屑灵优化方干预银屑病血瘀证患者尿液代谢机制研究. 广州中医药大学. 硕士. 2012.
S212	Cui Yali, 2011	崔亚丽, 加味黄连解毒汤治疗寻常型银屑病临床研究. 黑龙江科技信息. 2011;28.
S213	Qiu Guangli, 2002	仇广礼, 银屑病的中医辩证施治(附 30 例报告). 实用医药杂志. 2002;19(2):
S214	Cheng Fenglan, 2005	程凤兰, 白疕 2 号加味治疗寻常型银屑病疗效观察. 辽宁中医杂志. 2005;32(2):
S215	Chen Zhongchun, 2004	陈忠春, 天花粉汤治疗寻常性银屑病 66 例. 四川中医. 2004;22(2):73–74.
S216	Chen Yaodong, 2008	陈跃东, 清热凉血汤治疗寻常型银屑病 78 例. 黑龙江中医药. 2008;37(1):18–19.
S217	Chen Weimei, 2005	陈维梅, 中药治疗寻常型银屑病 210 例. 吉林中医药. 2005;25(9):
S218	Chen Sufen, 1998	陈素芬, 自拟消银祛斑汤治疗寻常型银屑病 54 例. 广西中医药. 1998;(05):38–46.
S219	Chen Su, 1998	陈苏, 消银方治疗银屑病. 山东中医杂志. 1998;17(11):499–500.
S220	Chen Lifu, 1998	陈立富, 银屑病治验 1 例. 江西中医药. 1998;29(5): 62.
S221	Chen Hui, 2004	陈慧, 姜黄煎剂对银屑病皮损中 CD45RO, VEGF 和 iNOS 表达的影响. 中国中西医结合皮肤性病学杂志. 2004;3(4):
S222	Cao Xuehui, 2001	曹雪辉, 凉血解毒方治疗风热血燥型寻常型银屑病 86 例. 新中医. 2001;33(7):
S223	Cao Wenlun, 2009	曹文伦, 消风散加减治疗银屑病 147 例. 浙江中西医结合杂志. 2009;19(9):577–578.

(*Continued*)

(Continued)

Number	First Author, Year	Reference
S224	Cai Shien, 1992	蔡世恩, 复方大黄汤治疗寻常型银屑病 30 例. 河南中医. 1992;(05):241–242.
S225	Anonymous, 1985	Anonymous, "克银方"治疗银屑病的研究. 医学研究通讯. 1985;(02):54.
S226	Anonymous, 1976	Anonymous, 24 例银屑病的中医疗效观察. 武汉医学院学报. 1976;(02):112–114.
S227	Anonymous, 1976	Anonymous, 银屑 I 号治疗银屑病 255 例的临床观察. 天津医药. 1976;(11):555–557.
S228	Anonymous, 1976	Anonymous, 中药复方山豆根片治疗银屑病(附 69 例报告). 重庆医药. 1976;(05):24–26.
S229	Geng Lidong, 1998	耿立东, 赵纯修辨证治疗寻常型银屑病 140 例总结. 山东中医杂志. 1998;17(12):555–556.
S230	Cui Xiaoru, 1987	崔效如, 中药烟治愈顽固性银屑病 12 例. 山西中医. 1987;(05):22–23.
S231	Liu Jinlian, 1988	刘锦莲, 应用骆驼蓬总碱治疗银屑病 69 例疗效观察. 天津中医. 1988;(6):9–10.
S232	Zhu Lin, 2008	祝林, 张华, 段永建. 中药"消癣灵"治疗寻常型银屑病 85 例疗效观察. 右江医学. 2008;36(2):230–1.
S233	Liu Xiaojun, 2012	刘效筠, 石年, 陈用军. 冰黄软膏外用治疗寻常型稳定期银屑病临床疗效观察. 湖北中医杂志. 2012;34(6):46.
S234	Han Chunlei, 2006	韩春雷, 彭建梅, 叶笑好. 冰黄肤乐软膏联合氯倍他索霜治疗寻常型银屑病临床观察. 中国皮肤性病学杂志. 2006;20(2):123,5.
S235	Wang Haiyan, 2010	王海燕, 孙燕, 李雪松. 中西医结合治疗寻常型银屑病 42 例临床观察. 中国现代医生. 2010;(30):55,67.
S236	Liu Huanqiang, 2005	刘焕强. 银屑病外洗方药浴联合窄谱中波紫外线照射治疗寻常型银屑病 40 例疗效观察. 新中医. 2005;37(2).
S237	Hu Zefang, 2007	胡泽芳. 窄频 UVB 联合中药熏蒸治疗寻常型银屑病疗效观察. 现代医药卫生. 2007;23(1).
S238	Cui Bingnan, 2008	崔炳南, 孙永新, 刘瓦利, 廖桂兰. 窄谱中波紫外线联合愈银方药浴治疗寻常型银屑病疗效观察. 中国中西医结合杂志. 2008;28(4):355–7.

(Continued)

(Continued)

Number	First Author, Year	Reference
S239	Liu Taihua, 2008	刘太华, 刘德芳, 陈璐, 罗陈, 许泽娟. 乌附酊剂/乌附油剂联合窄谱中波紫外线照射治疗寻常性银屑病临床观察. 临床皮肤科杂志. 2008;37(12):814–5.
S240	Chen Guiyin, 2009	陈贵银, 黄茂. 皮肤外洗浸泡为主治疗寻常型银屑病80 例临床观察. 河北中医药学报. 2009;24(3):22–3.
S241	Zhang Chunmin, 2009	张春敏, 魏国, 张春红, 庞力, 史永俭, 蔡莹. 中药熏蒸联合紫外线照射治疗银屑病的疗效及对血清中Th1/Th2 型细胞因子的影响. 中华物理医学与康复杂志. 2009(7):491–2.
S242	Chen Hong, 2010	陈宏, 张建波, 文景爱. 中药熏蒸联合 nb-Uvb 照射治疗银屑病的疗效观察. 国际中医中药杂志. 2010;32(3):249,58.
S243	Luo Shaomiao, 2010	罗绍淼, 范敏, 苏禧, 苏敬泽, 王亚梅. Nb-Uvb 联合中药浴治疗寻常性银屑病的临床观察. 中华皮肤科杂志. 2010(4):284–5.
S244	Wu Luna, 2010	伍露娜, 黄莉宁, 薛汝增. 窄谱中波紫外线联合中药浴治疗寻常型银屑病的疗效观察和护理. 皮肤性病诊疗学杂志. 2010;17(3):242–4.
S245	Zhang Yusuo, 2010	张玉锁, 魏录萍. Nb-Uvb 联合中药治疗寻常型银屑病疗效观察. 中国麻风皮肤病杂志. 2010(11):815.
S246	Shi Xiuli, 2011	师秀利, 潘玉明, 马会云, 杨学芬. 窄谱中波紫外线联合中药药浴治疗寻常型银屑病的临床疗效观察. 中国激光医学杂志. 2011;20(5):314–7.
S247	Wang Zhixin, 2011	王哲新, 王慧娟, 于子红, 耿庆娜, 任雷生, 顿耿, *et al.* 中药药浴联合窄谱中波紫外线治疗寻常型银屑病疗效观察. 河南大学学报·医学版. 2011;30(3):226–7.
S248	Wu Bo, 2011	吴波, 陈孝顶, 夏丹, 陈莉, 路永红, 张大维, *et al.* 中药药浴联合窄谱中波紫外线治疗寻常性银屑病疗效观察. 中国中西医结合皮肤性病学杂志. 2011;10(5):304–5.
S249	Zhang Chunhong, 2011	张春红, 张春敏, 杜锡贤, 蔡莹. 中药熏蒸联合紫外线照射治疗寻常型银屑病的疗效观察. 中华物理医学与康复杂志. 2011;33(12):937–9.

(Continued)

(Continued)

Number	First Author, Year	Reference
S250	Zhao Wenqing, 2011	赵文青. 中药熏蒸联合窄谱中波紫外线照射治疗寻常型银屑病 40 例疗效观察. 中国美容医学. 2011;20(z3).
S251	Zhu Xicong, 2012	朱希聪, 叶冬桂, 张为, 林兰英. 窄谱中波紫外线联合中药汽疗治疗寻常性银屑病的疗效观察. 现代实用医学. 2012;24(8):878–9.
S252	Lin Yingu, 2006	林胤谷. 复方青黛油膏治疗银屑病的临床疗效评估. 成都中医药大学学报. 2006;29(2).
S253	Qi Lin, 2010	祁林, 刘丽芳. 润肤止痒乳剂治疗寻常型银屑病血虚风燥证 30 例. 河南中医. 2010;30(11):1099–100.
S254	Tian Demao, 2002	田德茂, 王永彬, 周启东, 于立玲. 银屑净软膏外治寻常型银屑病临床研究. 中华临床新医学. 2002;2(12):1106–7.
S255	Cao Hongwei, 2008	曹鸿玮, 郑晓红, 王瑞, 杨俊亚. 冰黄肤乐软膏联合奥深软膏治疗寻常型银屑病临床疗效观察. 四川中医. 2008;26(11):96–7.
S256	Wang Jie, 2010	王洁, 邓长明, 李洁. 中药药浴联合窄谱中波紫外线治疗银屑病的疗效观察. 西部医学. 2010;22(12):2304–5.
S257	Cheng Lixue, 2011	程丽雪, 罗莉, 黄长松, 阮爱星. 中药药浴治疗中重度寻常型银屑病临床观察. 光明中医. 2011;26(5):938–40.
S258	Gong Zhiping, 2007	龚致平. 阿维 A 配合中药药浴治疗寻常型银屑病 96 例临床观察. 云南中医中药杂志. 2007;28(12).
S259	Sun Zejun, 2010	孙泽军, 米新陵, 时万杰, 华伟, 李凡. 中医药浴联合窄谱中波紫外线照射治疗寻常型银屑病的临床疗效观察. 当代医学. 2010;16(30):152–3.
S260	Wei Guo, 2008	魏国, 岳春雯, 张春敏, 刘瑛, 马冬梅 and 亓同刚, 银屑灵熏剂蒸汽治疗对寻常型银屑病外周血单个核细胞表达 T-bet, GATA-3 蛋白水平的影. 中国中西医结合杂志. 2008;28(12):1118–1120.
S261	Wang Enyin, 1999	王恩银, 银屑膏的制备与临床应用. 中国民间疗法. 1999;(05):36–37.
S262	Sun Lizhong, 1998	孙立忠 and 武瑞美, 银屑膏治疗银屑病 62 例. 湖南中医杂志. 1998;(05):35.

(Continued)

(Continued)

Number	First Author, Year	Reference
S263	Min Zhongsheng, 2004	闵仲生, 中药汽疗治疗寻常型银屑病的临床疗效观察及实验研究. 中国农村医学杂志. 2004;2(1):
S264	Ji Jun, 1989	纪钧, 张卫华, 王军 and 张友海, 消银油治疗银屑病 65 例. 辽宁中医杂志. 1989;(05):27–30.
S265	Du Xixian, 1999	杜锡贤, 袁玮, 汪五清, 刘翠娥 and 寇树堂, 镇银膏外治寻常型银屑病的临床与实验研究. 山东中医药大学学报. 1999;23(3):199–200.
S266	Du Xixian, 1999	杜锡贤, 镇银膏外治寻常型银屑病 105 例疗效观察. 中国医药学报. 1999;14(3):
S267	Yang Hengyu, 1991	杨恒裕, 中药填脐疗法治疗银屑病 106 例疗效观察. 北京中医学院学报. 1991;14(1):35.
S268	Jerner B, 1997	Jerner B, Skogh M, Vahlquist A. A controlled trial of acupuncture in psoriasis: no convincing effect. Acta dermato-venereologica. 1997 Mar;77(2): 154–6. PubMed PMID: 9111831. Epub 1997/03/01.
S269	Wu Jiaping, 2011	吴家萍, 谷世喆. 针灸治疗寻常型银屑病 30 例临床随机对照观察. 针刺研究. 2011;36(1):62–5.
S270	Wang Yuan, 2005	王元, 四时针刺与银屑病的相关研究. 针灸临床杂志. 2005, 21(3):
S271	Song Xuming, 2006	宋旭明, 隔蒜灸加针刺对寻常型银屑病疗效及相关细胞因子基因表达影响的研究. 成都中医药大学. 硕士. 2006.
S272	Liang Jingtao, 2007	梁静涛, 针刺背俞穴辅以局部灸法治疗银屑病的疗效观察. 四川中医. 2007;25(5):
S273	Chi Zhenrong, 1992	迟振荣, 王秀春 and 曲如花, 激光穴位照射治疗银屑病 62 例. 山东中医杂志. 1992;(01):27.
S274	Zhang Huicheng, 2011	张成会, 李斌, 丰靓, 姚尚萍 and 刘红霞, 中医特色外治疗法对寻常型斑块状银屑病的临床疗效观察. 中华中医药杂志. 2011;26(10): 2470–2472.

Glossary

Psoriasis Monograph
Glossary of Terms

Glossary of Terms	Acronym	Definition	Reference
95% confidence interval	95% CI	A measure of the uncertainty around the main finding of a statistical analysis. Estimates of unknown quantities, such as the odds ratio comparing an experimental intervention with a control, are usually presented as a point estimate and a 95% confidence interval. This means that if someone were to keep repeating a study in other samples from the same population, 95% of the confidence intervals from those studies would contain the true value of the unknown quantity. Alternatives to 95%, such as 90% and 99% confidence intervals, are sometimes used. Wider intervals indicate lower precision; narrow intervals, greater precision.	http://handbook.cochrane.org/
Acupressure	—	Application of pressure to acupuncture points.	—
Acupuncture	—	The insertion of needles into humans or animals for its methods or remedial purposes.	WHO International Standard Terminologies of Traditional Medicine in the Western Pacific Region. World Health Organisation, 2007.

Acupuncture point injection therapy	—	Combined therapy of acupuncture and medication by which liquid medicine is injected into the acupuncture point.	WHO International Standard Terminologies of Traditional Medicine in the Western Pacific Region. World Health Organisation, 2007.
Allied and Complementary Medicine Database	AMED	Alternative medicine bibliographic database.	https://www.ebscohost.com/academic/AMED-The-Allied-and-Complementary-Medicine-Database
Australian New Zealand Clinical Trial Registry	ANZCTR	Clinical Trial Registry.	http://www.anzctr.org.au/
Body Surface Area	BSA	Measured or calculated surface area of skin lesions.	Menter A, Gottlieb A, Feldman SR, van Voorhees AS, Leonardi CL, Gordon KB, *et al.* (2008) Guidelines of care for the management of psoriasis and psoriatic arthritis: Section 1. Overview of psoriasis and guidelines of care for the treatment of psoriasis with biologics. *J Am Acad Dermatol* **58**(5): 826–850.

(Continued)

(Continued)

Psoriasis Monograph Glossary of Terms	Acronym	Definition	Reference
China National Knowledge Infrastructure	CNKI	Chinese-language bibliographic database.	www.cnki.net
Chinese Biomedical Literature database	CBM	Chinese-language bibliographic database.	https://cbmwww.imicams. ac.cn
Chinese Clinical Trial Registry	ChiCTR	Clinical Trial Registry.	http://www.chictr.org
Chinese herbal medicine	CHM	Chinese herbal medicine.	—
Chinese medicine	CM	—	—
Chongqing VIP Information Company	CQVIP	Chinese-language bibliographic database.	http://www.cqvip.com
ClinicalTrials.gov	—	Clinical Trial Registry.	https://clinicaltrials.gov/
Cochrane Central Register of Controlled Trials	CENTRAL	Bibliographic database that provides a highly concentrated source of reports of randomised controlled trials.	http://community.cochrane. org/editorial-and-publishing-policy-resource/ cochrane-central-register-controlled-trials-central
Combination therapies	—	Two or more Chinese medicines from different therapy groups (CHM, acupuncture therapies or other CM therapies) administered together.	—

Term	Abbreviation	Definition	Source
Cumulative Index of Nursing and Allied Health Literature	CINAHL	Bibliographic database.	https://www.ebscohost.com/nursing/about
Cupping	—	Suction by using a vaccumised cup or jar.	WHO International Standard Terminologies of Traditional Medicine in the Western Pacific Region. World Health Organisation, 2007.
Dermatology Life Quality Index	DLQI	A measure of quality of life related to dermatological conditions.	Guidelines of care for the management of psoriasis and psoriatic arthritis
Effect size	—	A generic term for the estimate of effect of treatment for a study.	http://handbook.cochrane.org/
Effective rate	—	A measure of the proportion of participants who achieved an improvement, as outlined in the section on clinical evidence.	—
Electro-acupuncture	—	Electric stimulation of the needle following insertion.	WHO International Standard Terminologies of Traditional Medicine in the Western Pacific Region. World Health Organisation, 2007.
EU Clinical Trials Register	EU-CTR	Clinical Trial Registry.	https://www.clinicaltrialsregister.eu

(Continued)

(Continued)

Psoriasis Monograph Glossary of Terms	Acronym	Definition	Reference
Excerpta Medica dataBASE	Embase	Bibliographic database.	http://www.elsevier.com/solutions/embase
Grading of Recommendations Assessment, Development and Evaluation	GRADE	Approach to grading quality of evidence and strength of recommendations.	http://www.gradeworkinggroup.org/
Health-Related Quality of Life	HRQoL	A conceptual or operational measurement that is commonly used in the healthcare setting as a means to assess the impact of disease on the person.	Anderson DM. (2012) *Mosby's Dictionary of Medicine, Nursing & Health Professions.* Elsevier Health Sciences/Mosby, St. Louis, MO.
Heterogeneity	—	1. Used in a general sense to describe the variation in, or diversity of, participants, interventions, and measurement of outcomes across a set of studies, or the variation in internal validity of those studies. 2. Used specifically, as statistical heterogeneity, to describe the degree of variation in the effect estimates from a set of studies. Also used to indicate the presence of variability among studies beyond the amount expected due solely to the play of chance.	http://handbook.cochrane.org/

Term	Abbreviation	Definition	Source
Homogeneity	—	1. Used in a general sense to mean that the participants, interventions, and measurement of outcomes are similar across a set of studies. 2. Used specifically to describe the effect estimates from a set of studies where they do not vary more than would be expected by chance.	http://handbook.cochrane.org/
I^2	—	A measure of study heterogeneity, indicates the percentage of variance in a meta-analysis.	http://handbook.cochrane.org/
Intravenous	IV	Administered into a vein.	—
Koebner's phenomenon	—	The Koebner phenomenon, also called the 'Koebner response' or the 'isomorphic response', refers to skin lesions appearing on lines of trauma. It may result from either a linear exposure or irritation.	Anderson DM. (2012) *Mosby's Dictionary of Medicine, Nursing & Health Professions.* Elsevier Health Sciences/Mosby, St. Louis, MO.
Mean difference	MD	In meta-analysis: A method used to combine measures on continuous scales, where the mean, standard deviation and sample size in each group are known. The weight given to the difference in means from each study (e.g. how much influence each study has on the overall results of the meta-analysis) is determined by the precision of its estimate of effect and, in the statistical software in RevMan and the Cochrane Database of Systematic Reviews, is equal to the inverse of the variance. This method assumes that all of the trials have measured the outcome on the same scale.	http://handbook.cochrane.org/

(Continued)

133

(*Continued*)

Psoriasis Monograph Glossary of Terms	Acronym	Definition	Reference
Meta-analysis	—	The use of statistical techniques in a systematic review to integrate the results of included studies. Sometimes misused as a synonym for systematic reviews, where the review includes a meta-analysis.	—
Methotrexate	MTX	—	—
Moxibustion	—	A therapeutic procedure involving ignited material (usually moxa) to apply heat to certain points or areas of the body surface for curing disease through regulation of the function of meridians/channels and visceral organs.	WHO International Standard Terminologies of Traditional Medicine in the Western Pacific Region. World Health Organisation, 2007.
Narrowband UVB	NB-UVB	Narrowband UVB rays.	Menter A, Gottlieb A, Feldman SR, van Voorhees AS, Leonardi CL, *et al.* (2008) Guidelines of care for the management of psoriasis and psoriatic arthritis. *J Am Acad Dermatol* **58**(5): 826–850.
Noncontrolled studies	—	Observations made on individuals, usually receiving the same intervention, before and after an intervention but with no control group.	http://handbook.cochrane.org/

Non-randomised controlled trials	CCTs	An experimental study in which people are allocated to different interventions using methods that are not random.	http://handbook.cochrane.org/
Other Chinese medicine therapies	—	Other Chinese medicine therapies include all traditional therapies except Chinese herbal medicine and acupuncture, such as tuina and cupping.	—
PASI reduction 50%	PASI 50	A 50% reduction of PASI score.	Menter A, Gottlieb A, Feldman SR, van Voorhees AS, Leonardi CL, *et al.* (2008) Guidelines of care for the management of psoriasis and psoriatic arthritis. *J Am Acad Dermatol* **58**(5): 826–850.
PASI reduction 60%	PASI 60	A 60% reduction of PASI score.	Menter A, Gottlieb A, Feldman SR, van Voorhees AS, Leonardi CL, *et al.* (2008) Guidelines of care for the management of psoriasis and psoriatic arthritis. *J Am Acad Dermatol* **58**(5): 826–850.

(Continued)

(Continued)

Psoriasis Monograph Glossary of Terms	Acronym	Definition	Reference
PASI reduction 75%	PASI 75	A 75% reduction of PASI score.	Menter A, Gottlieb A, Feldman SR, van Voorhees AS, Leonardi CL, et al. (2008) Guidelines of care for the management of psoriasis and psoriatic arthritis. *J Am Acad Dermatol* **58**(5): 826–850.
Physicians Global Assessment	PGA	—	Menter A, Gottlieb A, Feldman SR, van Voorhees AS, Leonardi CL, et al. (2008) Guidelines of care for the management of psoriasis and psoriatic arthritis. *J Am Acad Dermatol* **58**(5): 826–850.
Psoralens followed by UVA phototherapy	PUVA	Administration of psoralens followed by UVA phototherapy.	Menter A, Gottlieb A, Feldman SR, van Voorhees AS, Leonardi CL, et al. (2008) Guidelines of care for the management of psoriasis and psoriatic arthritis. *J Am Acad Dermatol* **58**(5): 826–850.

Term	Abbrev.	Definition	Reference
Psoriasis Area and Severity Index	PASI	A measure of overall psoriasis severity and coverage.	Menter A, Gottlieb A, Feldman SR, van Voorhees AS, Leonardi CL, et al. (2008) Guidelines of care for the management of psoriasis and psoriatic arthritis. *J Am Acad Dermatol* **58**(5): 826–850.
PubMed	PubMed	Bibliographic database.	http://www.ncbi.nlm.nih.gov/pubmed
Randomised controlled trial	RCT	—	—
Risk of bias	—	Assessment of clinical trials to indicate if results may overestimate or underestimate the true effect because of bias in study design or reporting.	http://handbook.cochrane.org/
Risk ratio	RR	The ratio of risks in two groups. In intervention studies, it is the ratio of the risk in the intervention group to the risk in the control group. A risk ratio of one indicates no difference between comparison groups. For undesirable outcomes, a risk ratio that is less than one indicates that the intervention was effective in reducing the risk of that outcome.	http://handbook.cochrane.org/

(Continued)

137

(Continued)

Psoriasis Monograph Glossary of Terms	Acronym	Definition	Reference
Summary of findings	SOF	Presentation of results and rating the quality of evidence based on the GRADE approach.	http://www.gradeworkinggroup.org/
Tumour necrosis factor-α	TNF-α	A cytokine that is toxic to cancer cells and activates other leukocytes. It causes profound metabolic effects that include inflammatory responses, pyrexia and weight loss leading to cachexia.	Anderson DM. (2012) *Mosby's Dictionary of Medicine, Nursing & Health Professions.* Elsevier Health Sciences/ Mosby, St. Louis, MO.
Ultraviolet A	UVA	Ultraviolet A (long-wave) rays.	—
Ultraviolet B	UVB	Ultraviolet B (short-wave) rays.	—
Wanfang database	Wanfang	Chinese-language bibliographic database.	www.wanfangdata.com
World Health Organisation	WHO	The WHO is the directing and coordinating authority for health within the United Nations system. It is responsible for providing leadership on global health matters, shaping the health research agenda, setting norms and standards, articulating evidence-based policy options, providing technical support to countries and monitoring and assessing health trends.	http://www.who.int/about/en/

| Zhong Hua Yi Dian | ZHYD | The *Zhong Hua Yi Dian* (ZHYD) or *'Encyclopaedia of Traditional Chinese Medicine'* is a comprehensive series of electronic books on compact disk. The collection was put together by the Hunan electronic and audio-visual publishing house. It is the largest collection of Chinese electronic books and includes the major Chinese ancient works, many of which are from rare manuscripts and are the only existing copies. These books cover the period from ancient times upto the period of the Republic of China (1911–1948). | Hu R. (ed.), (2000) *Encyclopaedia of Traditional Chinese Medicine* 《中华医典》, 4th ed., Hunan Electronic and Audio-Visual Publishing House, Chengsha. |

Index

PASI, 5, 8, 9, 41, 42, 52, 53, 55, 57, 62, 64, 66, 69, 70, 92, 93, 96, 99, 135, 136, 137

phototherapy, 6, 7, 9, 35, 45, 47, 48, 53, 55, 61, 62, 64, 66, 70, 99, 136

plaque psoriasis, 1, 2, 6, 7, 9

psoriasis, 1–9, 13–15, 17–19, 21–27, 29, 30, 33, 35, 36, 41, 45–47, 50, 57, 61, 62, 66, 68–71, 73–75, 77, 80–82, 89, 90, 93–99, 102–105, 107, 126, 128, 129, 131, 134–137

randomised controlled trials, 46, 47, 50, 63, 90, 92, 95, 105

risk of bias, 36, 50, 63, 92

safety, 45, 61, 68, 89, 90, 94, 102

She shi, 23–27, 29, 97, 98, 103

Systematic Review, 33, 34, 39, 45, 89, 90

vulgaris, 1–3, 6–9, 45, 47, 50, 57, 61, 62, 66, 68–71, 73, 82, 89, 90, 93, 94, 97–99, 102–105

wound healing, 73, 78, 79

Zhong Hua Yi Dian, 21

www.ingramcontent.com/pod-product-compliance
Lightning Source LLC
Chambersburg PA
CBHW061252220326
41599CB00028B/5625